PRAISE FOR THE DOCTOR

Modern western science often defines
Ayurveda teaches that health is physi... ... emotional balance and
integration. In this treasure of a book, Sunita Passi brilliantly guides us
to an even deeper space of healing - where we are empowered to awaken
our innate wholeness. Through every magnificent page of this transformational journey, she reveals timeless truths, inspires us to make more
conscious choices, and lays out the blueprint for thriving in every aspect
of our life.

**Davidji, award-winning Author of Sacred Powers, globally recognized
Meditation teacher**

Sunita lives and breathes Ayurveda - and most importantly she brings it
to life in our chaotic world. This book is much more than a passive reading experience -in her no- nonsense style Sunita offers us the opportunity
to reflect on our own life's journey and the shifts needed to help us live
and be as we were born to do.

**Kate O Brien, bestselling Author of Your Middle Years and GLOW, Dieti-
tian and Yogi**

As a cardiologist I meet patients whose lives are damaged by a sick society. We can discover our best selves by reclaiming our birthright to make
wise choices about wellbeing. Sunita Passi is Ayurveda's brightest light,
and she's here to show you what this ancient healing art is about – your
body really does know best...if you know what it's telling you."

**Dr. Aseem Malhotra, Author of The Pioppi Diet, Cardiologist and
world-leading obesity expert**

This is more than a book sharing the powerful science of Ayurveda. As
well as an expert in her field, Sunita is truly grounded in our times. She
is showing us how modern and deeply needed Ayurveda's true principles
are if we want to heal ourselves and our planet and positively transform
todays healthcare systems.

**Dominique Antiglio, bestselling Author of The Life-Changing Power of
Sophrology, qualified Sophrologist and BeSophro Founder**

THE DOCTOR WON'T SEE YOU NOW

SEE YOU NOW

STAYING HEALTHY WHILE THE MEDICAL
SYSTEM IS RE-BOOTED

BY

SUNITA PASSI

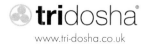

www.tri-dosha.co.uk

Published by Tri-Dosha Ltd. This title may be purchased in bulk for educational, business, fund-raising or sales promotional use. For ordering information, special discounts, or bulk purchases, please contact:
Admin, Tri-Dosha Ltd, NG3 6BG, UK.
E: info@tri-dosha.co.uk.
T: +44 (0) 115 752 2425.
W: www.tri-dosha.co.uk.

ISBN   978-1-3999-0611-1

9 781399 906111 >

Printed in the United Kingdom

I would like to dedicate this book to my parents, ultimately my greatest teachers. To India, for opening my heart and connecting me to the wisdom of Ayurveda. And finally to the many wellness therapists and skincare professionals without whose blessed support, wisdom and nurturing I would never have found my true purpose.

CONTENT

INTRODUCTION

What does health mean to you?
Is it the absence of illness?
The presence of wellbeing?
Our sense of who we are and how we
are changes over time.

As children, if we fall and graze ourselves, a parent's willingness to kiss it better can take away the pain. Or does it 'just' stop the child crying? If attention is part of what makes us feel valued or whole, then maybe that kiss really is doing something useful. Or maybe there's something chemical going on in mum's saliva, yet to be isolated and trademarked and sold to us as a product.

Already then, we have a few concepts involved in what being well involves:

- It's about more than our bodies.
- It involves how people engage with one another.
- It doesn't always require trained professionals and branded products.

Let's look at what the first of those bulletpoints shows when we put aside how easy the sentence sounds and think about what it implies. In other words:

- What does it even mean to say 'It's about more than our bodies'?

The fact we can even say something of that sort without people looking at us funny is an indication of the power of a sentence first uttered by a Frenchman in the 17th century:

Cogito ergo sum.

That's it in Latin at least, which is how the phrase appeared in the work of René Descartes. He wrote it in Latin because that's one way you can make things sound grander than they are, a gimmick the Catholic Church has long used to hoodwink people. In English we know those words as:

I think, therefore I am.

Sounds pretty good at first. But bear in mind, never trust a philosophy that works as a t-shirt slogan.

Let's ponder what's both being said, and not being said, in those words.

It makes thinking out to be the bees' knees in terms of human experience. Human, because there's an implicit suggestion we are the only species to think in a way that counts. And you can guess, since Descartes is a mighty thinker writing for other mighty thinkers, that when he refers to thought he means language.

Birdsong is certainly articulation. It's been shown to help people feel happy. Looked at more closely though, surely it's merely random warbling of no distinction. When did a lark last tell you a joke?

Just like that, making thought-in-the-form-of-words a bigger deal than other forms of pondering and expression, Descartes ruled out any animal that ever lived. They might not know Latin, but creatures can express awareness and make choices in many ways. That includes dolphins rescuing stranded swimmers, elephants gathering together in what seems very much like ceremony for a dead member of their herd, crows figuring out puzzles many people can't do.

Even putting animals aside, there are other problems with Descartes. One becomes apparent by rearranging his words:

I am, therefore I think.

Immediately we're in other territory. If existence precedes thinking, then maybe thought is just one aspect of something bigger. As for what that could be, how about:

I feel, therefore I am.

Let's go back to that toddler with the grazed knee, unable to distinguish between...

- the pain of the fall
- skin that's had a layer or two exposed
- a spot of blood
- the lamb she wanted to say hello to and grandad told her not to
- being more determined to befriend the lamb and running over to it
- the ground coming up and hitting her when she fell
- memories of other times she's not only failed to do what she wants but been punished for it
- hating lambs and needing right now that magic moment mum can provide with a kiss

It's fair to say there isn't a pill capable of doing all of the things in that precious moment of contact between mother and child.

You can create your own examples that involve other people and settings. Your own history will let you know life is woven together in ways that seem slippery. The twinge you got in your stomach for years when you dealt with an authority figure which stopped when you did aikido lessons. Migraines that seem to come up when you eat dairy products, whatever your cousin the optician says. That lump your doctor swears is benign but looks just like one your father and grandfather had in the same place, who died of the same unidentified cause.

You can't easily unpick one person from another, the places they live and work, and the conditions in which they do both. At which point we're unavoidably getting into politics. For instance, it's said both of African-Americans, and people from the Indian subcontinent living in the UK, that they are more prone to respiratory conditions. It's also the case that many who fit those descriptions live in busy urban areas where exhaust fumes make greater pollution a fact of daily life. Reducing carbon monoxide is a huge problem, and lethargy in dealing with it is linked to the political clout of the auto industry and oil companies. Easier to hand out asthma inhalers.

People struggling to make enough money to get by necessarily have less money to eat. Many cities aren't readily provided with sources of good quality calories for those on low incomes. Instead, fast food can become a norm that starts in childhood and can soon lead to obesity and its consequences. Breaking out of the habit – sugars and fats give a quick hit that feels like pleasure – isn't easy.

So when you turn up in a hospital, wheezing and overweight, what do the doctors do? Help you find better paid work in an area where there are less cars? That would be ridiculous, wouldn't it? Why? One serious plan to improve health in the UK is to develop a new sewage system. Proponents say it would have a bigger impact on public health than spending an equivalent amount on medical treatments as we understand them.

Time for another question:
What are we talking about, when we talk about health?

Usually, when those conversations come up, the NHS is part of the discussion if you're British. It's an incredible and rightly treasured institution. I was born in an NHS hospital, as were two of my siblings. Beautiful children born to friends have come into the world in one.

But something isn't working. Take a walk around the corridors of a hospital and you'll get some clues. Odds are there'll be several floors and many departments in the building – usually more than one building, because hospitals are big. You might take 10 minutes to find the room to talk with a specialist about your leg, who will send you another 10 minutes away to have blood taken for some tests. On the basis of the results you get to see another expert in an adjacent building who says you have gout which - guess what - they write papers about. Then go to a pharmacy back to pick up the tablets prescribed. Six weeks later you return. The tablets haven't helped. You see another consultant on a higher floor. They say the issue isn't gout, but uric acid crystal around joints very similar to the ones gout produces but not the same. And it can be cleared up with some other tablets. Which is a relief, because the gout medication was something you'd have been on for the rest of your life if that label had stuck, rather than being peeled off by a more perceptive doctor.

Follow the arrows around a hospital's seemingly infinite number of corridors, and to the rooms where you'll find out what's wrong and hopefully get a cure. Clearly the system could be made more efficient. Perhaps a patient's blood and leg could be sent to different departments simultaneously, while the head stays talking to a consultant? OK, exaggerating there. But with a point:

Maybe the parts don't matter more than the whole.
Maybe a better approach is to start with the patient in their entirety.

If what counts is a person's...everything, then the notion of health changes. Some things are more or less givens. Genetically you may be predisposed to diabetes. Whether you get it is another matter. Sometimes it's about diet, which potentially brings us back to class and recognising that a better lifestyle assumes choices based on good information and the resources to act on it. Working three jobs doesn't help with that. Diabetes can also result from shock. In either case, there are more and less effective ways to live with the condition. Notions of agency and discipline come into this: changing habits for the better is tricky, whatever the payoff. Especially in a culture where emotional needs are often satisfied not directly but in the form of baked goods, alcohol, or career status.

Media is complicit in this, sometimes overtly through advertising, and in other forms too. The appearance of impossibly buffed Hollywood actors drives traffic to plastic surgeons, where horrors are committed in the name of people feeling better about themselves. Instagram influencers dangle the prospect of fabulous lives attainable if you just buy the right stuff.

Facebook, with access to all your data, knows when you're at your most vulnerable and when to pop up that coupon for a pizza. And here's the thing:

We don't need fixing. We're not broken.

Can you imagine a society where people lived as if that was true?

You don't need to imagine. There are and have been examples throughout human history.

In traditional Chinese medicine, which addressed the whole person, community practitioners would be paid not for making people 'better', but for preventing illness in the first place. The same attitude was espoused by the esoteric British master Winston Churchill, who said that healthy citizens are a nation's greatest asset.

How we ended up in a situation where the NHS is less about delivering health services, than administering their delivery is not a matter for this book. If you know anyone who works for the NHS or has left because of the pressures they experienced even pre-covid, you may have some sense of what that means beyond your experience as a patient.

Vultures in the form of private American companies swoop over an organisation regarded as one of the finest accomplishments in human history. It may or may not be possible to realign the NHS with its original intentions. And there are signs of promise even within current changes: written online consultations about trivial matters allow GPs extra time to spend with patients who really do need longer 1:1 contact. But we can do more. And need to.

Many of the factors that go into whether someone has happier or less satisfying experiences of health can be affected with some simple changes, many inexpensive or even free:

- Drinking more water is a negligible cost.
- Getting outdoors not just for exercise, but to spend time in fresher air and around plants and trees…feels good because it is. Don't overthink it: that's how Descartes went wrong.
- Finding ways to unstress, destress, or whatever else might take that unpleasantness away… you'll never regret that.
- Experiencing joy matters. Whatever we're here for almost certainly doesn't involve spreadsheets and traffic jams. Find whatever makes you smile inside and do it more.

Medication and operations will always have an important part to play in how people experience healthcare. The assumption that they are the default is problematic. Some conditions are medicalised which never needed that setting. Mental health has provided many dismal examples over the years.

In 1850, Samuel Cartwright discovered a condition he called drapetomania, from the Greek drapetes meaning 'runaway slave'. Drapetomania was defined as "the disease causing Negroes to run away", the chief symptom of which was "absconding from service".

No concept there that an escapee may have every reason in the world to flee their chains. 'Crazy' these days equals whatever gets into the pages of the Diagnostic and Statistical Manual of Mental Disorders – the DSM - produced by the American Psychiatric Association. Admittedly, they have previously declared that homosexuality is a mental illness, though changed their minds in 1974.

The most recent edition of the DSM includes the alarming condition Oppositional Defiant Disorder. If your child or teenager exhibits frequent and persistent anger, irritability, arguing, defiance or vindictiveness toward you and other authority figures, he or she may have oppositional defiant disorder. As such they may require treatment, possibly including medication.

Ask yourself how many children or teenagers you've come across who that description doesn't fit at least some of the time. It's pretty much the job description for an adolescent. You may have been a feisty one yourself. If not, there's never been a better time for well-motivated exuberant defiance than now, or a cause more important than taking more of your life back into your own hands. And it can start as simply as eating more fresh fruit and veg.

I'm passionate about these matters because they're at the core of the person I've become and have defined so much of what I've done for two decades.

Some years ago, I was a successful business journalist. A lot of my time was spent on planes and in hotels, a jetset lifestyle interviewing business founders and leaders, many experiencing considerable success.

The boss of the agency I worked with was a vibrant example of someone whose working life had brought them fulfilment and joy and allowed them to do what mattered in her own life and be of benefit to others. Another who made a big impression had been born in the Philippines, built up a flourishing business over 15 years, and enjoyed time at her flats in Rome (opera close by) and Paris (where she painted). Amazing people with rich multi-faceted lives.

Others experience satisfaction without riches. Or find getting by a grind, which of course it can be for many. And others still achieve wealth without finding it rewarding.

The best bit of that discomfort, the gap between what you're told and what you feel? You've probably sensed it for a good while now. You're among friends. Anyone who's got this far into these pages is nodding the same way you are, whether that's a visible head movement, a voice saying you're reading something more or less true, or the feeling that this book is one you'll be telling friends about.

Anyway, I crashed and burned in India. Of all the countries in all the world, I chose the land of my ancestors to be put back together again. That choice had little to do with the person I knew as myself at the time. Me now sees the sense of it all a whole new way.

The place itself didn't do the healing. Not on its own at least, glad of that connection as I was. Instead, I experienced something arising from that land and its people: the ancient system of Ayurveda. Thousands of years of wisdom about how body and nutrition and breathing and sleep and herbs. A superficially simple but infinitely rich way of understanding how people get to be who they are which takes temperament and physique into account. Straightforward and joyous ways to connect with self and more through meditation. A profound understanding of the body articulated through yoga and massage. And an underlying ethos shared with traditional Chinese medicine: treat yourself and others right to begin with, and they and you won't need 'fixing' in any form.

None of this would have been possible had the architects of Ayurveda been so self-satisfied as to mistake 'I think, therefore I am' for more than a passing brainfart.

Ayurveda became my life. I soaked up trainings, and in doing so realised their resonance went back to my earliest years. Without being aware of it, fragments of Ayurvedic practice had made their way into my childhood thanks to my grandfather, who I had not realised was an accomplished healer in the tradition.

What remained was to bring my business knowhow to turn Ayurveda's elegant wisdom into an economically effective means of enabling people to become kinder to themselves and those in their lives. Really, that's what a lot of this boils down to. There are principles, there is knowledge, and technique. But at heart, it's about heart.

I grew my business Tri-Dosha. Sometimes it seems it grew itself. But I know how much work I've put into it. Those years speaking with CEOs, managing directors, and entrepreneurs taught me a lot about their kind of success and how it allowed them to contribute personally and socially, while also reflecting on the signs of deep dissatisfaction some exhibited. There were certainly lessons to be learned about building a commercially effective enterprise, and I approached that in the spirit of my new understandings.

As well as offering products made in the traditional ways and even the same locations my grandfather grew plants he made treatments with, I worked with retailers to create products suited to their brands, trained more than 1200 people as Ayurvedic wellness therapists and practitioners and...lots more! It's been exhilarating throughout, and the sense at times has been that every step forward I make presents a future I get an increasing sense of. The best way I can articulate it is in the words of esteemed novelist and scriptwriter Neil Gaiman (Coraline, Good Omens, Sandman, etc). He's talking here about developing a story, recounted by fellow comics creator Dave Sim, and it's very much my experience of building Tri-Dosha:

"It's as if you're building a bridge, but you're not building a bridge sequentially, the way you have to do it in the physical world. The moment you start building it on this side, it starts growing from the other side. And you just start trying to predict where all the curlicues and whatnot are going to be, and all of a sudden one of them shows up, and you've got a chunk of the bridge about 30 feet out in mid-air that's about 15 feet higher than you thought it was supposed to be."

Tri-Dosha has plenty of curlicues and whatnot. Especially when, pre-covid, the business had a presence at Belvoir castle. Now, it's time for a different approach. To communicate with more people in new ways. That's part of the impetus for this book. And in reading it, if you too become motivated to consider health and the way it relates to the natural and social worlds, and how both are affected by the various insanities of our current ways of living, I will consider this return to text a success. Though business was my specialism as a journalist, in exploring it I trained in investigative journalism. You can look forward to some interesting questions in the chapters ahead, and surprising answers.

IT'S YOUR TURN

This book isn't designed as a passive experience. I want to use the themes and examples used in different sections to get you reflecting on your own history and shifts in your understanding of health over time. You might want to do that chapter by chapter, or on finishing the text. You do you.

With that in mind, these are prompts for some writing of your own – in these pages, in a journal, or in a digital form. Mostly but not always they occur at ends of chapters. Over the course of these pages, the idea is for you to get a richer sense of your shifting perceptions of wellbeing.

Feel free to use images as part of what you put down. Doodles, sketches, photos even. All can shed light, and sometimes a picture can capture something you either lack the right words for, or contains something which has a rightness beyond words.

Let's begin with some questions about childhood and health.

1. As a child, how were everyday ailments handled? Did some version of 'kiss it better' exist in your family?
2. Looking back, can you recall how and when that approach was used? What did you experience that would let you know it was time for that kind of reassurance? What would you call that experience now?
3. If you have children, is that something you now do with your own kids? When do you know it's called for, and how do they respond?
4. What is your recollection of early experiences of nurses, doctors, and dentists? Were they associated with relatives in hospital? How was that compared to your experience of a GP visit?
5. How did others in your family relate to health professionals? Were there stories that made you impressed, or scared? Growing up, did you know anyone working in health through your family? What impact did they make on you?

Thinking now about mental health...

1. Were you aware of people in or around your family with mental health issues? How were they spoken of, and how did you relate to

them?

2. Could you sense a difference between them and the other adults in your life? Was it a good difference or not?

3. Looking back, what would you say about the people you encountered with what we'd call mental health issues now? How much of what they experienced might have been a response to relationship breakup, work stress, or social pressures?

4. Have you had some kind of breakdown yourself? Was the support that you had useful or less so? Did you have a sense at the time what might be going on and were you able to get that across to people around you?

5. Was there a point you realised that the way you and the world were described didn't match your experience? How did that feel, and what did you do about it?

Looking at things from a social perspective...

1. Do you feel you were more or less fortunate in your upbringing? How has that affected your wellbeing and the choices you can make around it?

2. Did parental input and education create positive impressions of the kind of life you could lead? Were those impressions roughly accurate?

3. Where have you found role models in life? Are they in your family and social circle? In people you know through their lives and careers thanks to the impact they've made? Do they exist in fiction, myth, or religion?

4. If you'd been brought up in another culture, how do you imagine things might have been different? Would the you raised in California or Israel be broadly the same as the person you've become?

5. What do you take for granted about health and healthcare that you've had cause to reconsider over the years? How do you imagine those beliefs may need to change thinking to a decade ahead?

BIRTH PAINS

THE NHS

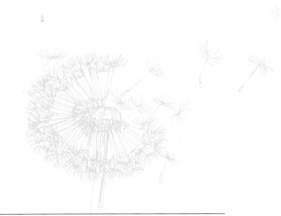

It would be fair to describe Britain's National Health Service as one of the wonders of the modern world. Soldiers who fought in World War Two returned home and had no intention of voting for Churchill. Strong wartime leader he may have been, but the qualities and presence required for that role were a world away from those required for social and economic reconstruction. Women too wanted to see a different nation – for themselves, and the children they'd be bringing up in a post-war birth boom.

Put all that together and you get the creation of the welfare state, from a template outlined in the 1942 Beveridge Report with healthcare for returning soldiers in mind. It was Aneurin Bevan, Minister for Health under Prime Minister Clement Attlee, who got to steer through the realities of that vision. What he encountered was a different kind of politics than the sort which brought Labour to power...

A lot of doctors would be needed to realise the dream Labour had in mind. That put the British Medical Association - the body representing the profession - in an interesting position. As such, there were times when they put the interests of their members over the government of the day. It's been the case since the BMA was formed in 1832. Later that decade they spoke against the Poor Law, noting its provisions were "insulting and degrading to the character of the medical profession as they were unjust and injurious to the poor." Note who comes first in the two groups listed...and doctors were far from poor.

All of that meant the BMA were wary about what Bevan could do to the comfortable situation they'd secured over the preceding century. How unimpressed were they? Doctors voted 10 to 1 against forming the health service. BMA members were particularly scathing about doctors as state employees with set salaries, flexing their muscles to retain payment based on the number of registered patients. Surgeries remained private businesses, now contracted to provide services by the NHS, which was frustrating for Bevan given the costs involved in making free healthcare for all possible.

Hard to imagine now, but in 1946 a former BMA chair noted the parliamentary bill to bring the NHS into being "looks to me uncommonly like the first step, and a big one, to national socialism as practiced in Germany." Churchill was of the same opinion.

COUNTERPOINT: 1

In 1959, Fidel Castro ensured things unfolded differently when he led his country's revolution and became Cuba's leader for life. Without a pressure group like the BMA and its stranglehold controlling the numbers in the medical profession, Castro rolled out a programme which as well as providing comprehensive and effective care for Cubans, trained thousands of additional health professionals. In the 2010s 50,000 were active, supporting people in developing countries, and creating benefits for those nations they wouldn't have experienced otherwise.

THE NHS EXPANDS

Over decades the NHS grew. Its sheer scale, coupled with committed and well-trained staff embracing methods that achieve unquestionable results, allows amazing things to happen. Since 1948, deaths by heart disease and strokes have fallen by 40%. That same year 20,000 died of tuberculosis. The 2016 figure was 196. More broadly, people are living longer: the mortality rate – effectively the likelihood that you will die in a given year - was significantly lower in 2015 than in the aftermath of WW2. The NHS won't be the only factor involved there (a fuller picture would include looking at diet, lifestyle, occupation, and more) but clearly healthcare is central to that progress.

And the NHS kept growing. As of September 2020 the service dealt with a million patients every 36 hours, all funded by taxpayers through income tax, national insurance, or VAT. Annual budget in 2019: £134 billion. Its exact size in people terms has varied over the years but has long hovered around the midpoint of the world's 10 biggest employers. Bigger than the Korean Army, smaller than America's, and in the ballpark of McDonald's with around 1.2 million employees, down from 1.5m in 2015.

Of that total, half have no medical qualifications. Which means whatever they're doing, not all are directly involved in making sick people healthy. For some reason we fail to identify ourselves with the USSR and Eastern European countries where crushing bureaucracy was long a source of dark humour, probably because of the merited reputation the NHS for being so brilliant for several generations of British families. Such sentimentalism gets in the way of a more considered response to the realities of the service.

If the NHS were an organism rather than an organisation it might be easier to see what the effect of such expansion has been. There's a word for what happens in a living being when its growth spirals out of control. When the proliferating cells are abnormal, that word is cancer.

What does abnormal mean? In this context, adding tiers of management designed to rein in the tendencies of a system to heal people in ways that over decades became costly, inefficient, and inconsistent. And the more systems to prevent such sprawl were installed, the greater the effort required to assert control became. Which is how the NHS became a bureaucracy on an unparalleled scale. Layers of new staff with a focus on tidy spreadsheets not patient bedsheets, soaking up money and cascading administrative systems taking up medical staff time, creating frustration for healthcare professionals and their patients alike.

The desire to get good value from the monies spent on the NHS has led to ridiculous results. How likely is it that a GP can assess the root cause of a patient's condition in the scope of a ten minute appointment? Even if they recognise their own inability to target it with precision, can their assumption about which specialist may be suited to deal with the situation be accurate on the basis of a fleeting meeting?

The NHS is a world wonder, unquestionably. And like the seven we know by that name, it's increasingly likely that it will soon be a thing of the past. The simple facts for that forecast are financial.

A VICTIM OF ITS OWN SUCCESS

If death by heart attacks and strokes are down thanks to the success of the NHS over decades, what are people suffering with instead? Increased longevity brings with it a greater prospect of dementia. And that has costs which ripple within and beyond the NHS.

Living longer with declining faculties can be a tragedy for families as well as individuals. And the financial aspects are various. More often than not, it's female relatives who will devote less time to paid work to care for ageing parents or aunts and uncles. That affects both household budgets, and the amount of tax they're putting into the NHS. And because those carers have time but lack all of the skills required to perform that care role effectively, support from taxpayer funded social support as well as health budgets is involved.

The lines between social and health care are inevitably blurred. The distinction has always been artificial. An individual's health depends on large part on being part of a functional community. And since the Industrial Revolution, when rural populations were lured into towns with the promise of better money and employers that would look after you and your family, things have changed considerably.

In that time, people have become viewed less as citizens than consumers. Taken from the land we lived on and tended to a few generations ago, we now experience food less as something to be grown and enjoyed, than fuel to be consumed at either end of a working day chosen because of its branding. And however appealing branding may be, it doesn't guarantee the contents of a packet or tin are as wholesome as what the imagery of ads and labels implies. Diabetes and obesity are often associated with branded foods – and are major contributors to developing Alzheimer's. Part of why we like such overly sugary and/or salted foods is the quick hit they provide – a temporary release from the stresses involved in living and working in a town where on top of a demanding job you could be juggling life with a partner, kids, and a parent in a care home.

In 2018 a report suggested that to stay on top of its duties, the NHS would need to bring in more tax revenues, an extra £2000 annually per household. That's a lot of money. Niall Dickinson, chief executive of the NHS Confederation, explained why he believed it was essential. "Over the next 15 years in the UK, there will be four million more people over 65, and the prospect of a 40% increase in hospital admissions and further large increases in the number of people with numerous long-term conditions."

What Dickinson was pointing to was true enough. But take a closer look. The report was conducted by the Institute for Fiscal Studies. Note the emphasis on money. Their whole remit is around notions of economic value as perceived through a narrow lens. Money savings good, waste bad. Sounds great, but these matters become tricky to assess when humans living in community are assessed. And the IFS is much more on the side of big business and wealth, cautioning that taxing the rich and corporations has its limits. Which may well explain why it's more in favour of ground level citizens picking up the tab. Cynically, you could even suggest that the IFS had their eye on a longer game, one that would increase corporate wealth and power.

COUNTERPOINT: 2

America's radical Black Panther movement are mainly thought of as leather-jacketed gun-toting African-Americans in the 1960s and 70s. They were founded in 1966 owing to widespread experiences of prejudice and worse from the police. Two years later they started Peoples Free Medical Clinics due to discrimination in the medical system and some hospitals. Their clinics provided screening for sickle cell anaemia, instrumental in the condition's wider recognition.

In 1970, Panthers began providing free breakfasts for children. By addressing issues of poverty and community, the Panthers made clear that food economics are just as much part of the bigger picture of healthcare as well-funded hi-tech facilities that profit businesses in and around pharma. Opposition came in various forms. If you were lucky, you'd experience passive-aggressive bureaucracy. Less fortunate Panther operations were directly attacked by police or undermined by FBI operations.

THERE'S GOLD IN THEM THERE PILLS

The NHS is internationally admired. An American study rated it as the world's best. It's certainly a hugely impressive system. And for all its bloat and expense, it's actually pretty efficient – when compared to what happens for Americans.

A key point that advocates of the US health insurance model make is that it keeps government in its place. Meaning, out of the affairs of its citizens. The Black Panther example makes clear things aren't quite that simple. Especially when citizens wish to take healthcare into their own hands, depriving god-fearing corporations of their right to profit from the public.

The argument for keeping American health the way it has been is its efficiency: corporations know all about money, after all. From that perspective, the 8% of UK money that the government spent on the NHS in 2019 is an abomination. The comparable figure for the States was a slimline...8.1%. Which can't be right, surely...? Except that it is. Pretty much the same figure was spent on private health in America, making for a total of 16.2% of the nation's money going on a ridiculously broken system. Much of that money gets nowhere near patients or health professionals. It's in the hands of the insurance industry, and America has a curiously partisan attitude about protecting the ability of businesses to make money...

Johnson & Johnson baby powder is used by women worldwide. It's possible that the ovarian cancer 22 American women developed when they used it had something to do with the product. A court was convinced enough by the possibility to award those affected a sum totalling $4.7 bn in 2018. Johnson & Johnson didn't believe that was fair, so fought to reduce that settlement to $2.1 bn, and whittled down the plaintiffs to 20. Further pondering by the company resulted in them realising they'd rather not pay compensation at all in a June 2021 case, for reasons more clear to lawyers than anyone who might have reason to believe baby powder containing asbestos caused their cancer. The company's case was dismissed by the Supreme Court.

Businesses looking to profit have a few options available to them. One is to innovate in useful ways. But the odds are uncertain, and it takes a long time. Anyway, there's more money to be made through gaming the systems by which money is now created. That mode of capitalism has been increasingly prevalent since 2008, when the banks and their allies responsible for a global economic crash received no meaningful penalties for their misbehaviours, and governments nervously agreed to their demands to be bailed out.

At that point, all bets were off. The years since have shown that time and again. Desire to innovate has been replaced by the desire to disrupt. And disruption has no care for the trail it leaves behind, which makes it unsurprising that the NHS has been eyed up by those who see it as a source of profit shamefully hogged by the British public in need of a new home with those seeking to create more billions. The moneys they believe are rightfully theirs will come from data. Your data.

INFORMATION IS EVERYTHING

You've probably heard the expression 'Information is the new oil'. Meaning, that's where money gets made these days. The words take me to a banner I saw in a photo of people protesting America's involvement in Iraq for access to its oil fields. The banner read 'How did our oil get under their soil?'.
Where we are at this point with the NHS, is the distinct probability that patient data will be making money for its new custodians without you seeing any of it or being told much if anything about how that money is cooked up. 'Custodians' suggests rather more care with information that could include details of your sexual history, mental health episodes, and traumas, than you would ever willingly share with businesses whose sole purpose is to maximise profit.

The NHS is already in what seems very much like a closing-down sale. Spending on services provided by private companies increased by 14% between 2014 and 2019/20, when the figure totalled £9.7 billion. During the same period, budgets for the NHS overall grew at a slower rate (1.4% on average from 2009/10 to 2018/19) than the average 3.7% annual increase since the service was founded.

While some of those figures may well have represented better expenditure, it's hard not to be left with the assumption that there's been a concerted drive to spend more with private providers. The £9.7 billion expenditure in 2019/20 omits several categories of health provision:

- Primary care (GPs, pharmacies, dentists, opticians)
- Local authorities
- Voluntary and not-for-profit

Estimates of what that represents in terms of NHS expenditure suggest that in total 25% of NHS spending goes to the private sector.

In addition, there are covid-specific payments, which seem to have a way of getting to people with close ties to the government. £37bn was spent on a Test & Trace system that doesn't do either of those tasks very well, and was more expensive to deliver than NASA getting a vehicle to wander around the surface of Mars. At least that technology sent us pictures to look at.

Facebook demonstrated that if you're not paying for a product, then you yourself are the product. One with years of data that advertisers use to target you based on information about everything from your holiday choices to musical preferences and time of maximum vulnerability to ordering a pizza when reminded about an ex by a new photo of them looking great.

If you're not concerned about what NHS health data could be used for, you need to be. Not least because of the service's relationship with Palantir, an American information tech firm with strong CIA connections brought in by the government to work with data at the time covid kicked off. Opposition to Palantir may yet mean the company doesn't get to make use of NHS data to the extent perhaps scoped out. Let's hope so. In the States, it was information provided by the company – whose expertise is bringing facts from multiple sources together – that allowed children to be separated from their parents when the Trump administration was targeting people who'd come to America undocumented. It's a world away from the NHS that brings babies into the world every year and helps give them a better start in life than their parents had.

COUNTERPOINT: 3

In China centuries ago, doctors were paid not for the patients that they were obliged to work with to heal, but to prevent people in their communities becoming ill in the first place. Their ethos took in diet and exercise and considered the whole person rather than just their symptoms. Any information gathered had a context to the individual, their family, the fields and season and more.

It wasn't just the Chinese who took that kind of holistic approach to wellbeing. In India, families across the country benefitted from the centuries of knowledge contained within the system we call Ayurveda. And the principles it embodies can be applied for yourself and those you know to contribute vitally to your state of physical, mental, and emotional happiness. Hoarding data can mean power and wealth to some, but the timeless wisdom of Ayurveda is more truly about freedom and connection.

IT'S YOUR TURN

Let's take a look at the role the NHS has played in your life, and your family's and community's, over time. As before, feel free to use diagrams and photos or anything else that might help. Maybe it would be good to chat with relatives for some info, too.

1. When did you first become aware of the National Health Service? Did you already have prior medical experience and found out it came from the NHS later?
2. How was the NHS talked about in stories shared by family members? Something to be loved and fought for? A bureaucracy that makes it hard for people to get what they need? What were the range of stories you heard?
3. Do you have a sense of those stories changing over time? Can you distinguish between family experiences and what you came across through the media?
4. How have portrayals of the health service in BBC dramas such as Casualty, Holby City, Doctors, Angels and Call the Midwife shaped your and your family's view of the NHS?
5. What about how hospitals and doctors and nurses were depicted in Carry On films? Did they seem to have a truth to them, and how was it different to what was seen in the tv dramas?
6. Do you know people who work in the NHS? What do they say about it now versus how it was when they started? How about people who used to work there?
7. What's your sense of what works well in the NHS and what doesn't?

8. Draw the NHS. Is it an animal? A factory? An orchestra? A vehicle? A circus? Have fun coming up with an image (maybe several) that captures the ups and downs and duration of your experience.
9. How does your experience of alternative and complementary health differ from what you've had with the NHS?

CHER ∧ND CHER ∧LIKE

MY JOURNEY

Of all the guides and healers I've worked with, the most transformational has been Cher. Yes, the singer and actress. True, she's also been called a Goddess of Pop, and her super-catchy song Believe delivers an uplifting message in 4 minutes. But personal transformation isn't what most people would think of if she comes to mind.

How it happened was through going to an ashram in 2002. If you're unfamiliar with the term, an ashram is a place dedicated to people gathering there achieving their desires. Everyone brings what they bring, whether it's healing trauma, finding purpose in life, or making material progress. Often an ashram is led by a teacher or guru of some sort. The methods could include meditation classes, exercise, and there's a lot to be said for the supportive atmosphere of being among a community of people sharing the experience. And being well fed in an amazing place, with a stunning green forest to wander in, is always welcome. All of which made the ashram a place conducive to stepping outside your boundaries...

There was a room we called the Buddha hall. And one thing we did was a laughing meditation. We all carry stress and pain with us in various forms. You might recall that old saying about laughter being the best medicine. There are reasons for that. I discovered them. I did Believe.

Laughing is a liberation. Think why we go to see a show by a comedian.

Yes, they're making their sharp observations about matters of the day, unpicking hypocrisies and highlighting nonsense in whatever form it appears. Or falling about in front of us, getting things wrong to remind us that we're all fools and clowns. Whatever's going on, it involves more than sitting in a room with a bunch of strangers moving your shoulders up and down and wheezing with the hilarity of what the person on stage is saying and doing.

A word that can be useful here is *catharsis*, which is to do with restoring balance. The process can combine the physical, mental, emotional, as woven from past through to now and shape our sense of the future. Catharsis pretty much contains the word arse. A good rule of thumb when remembering catharsis is to think *laughing your arse off*.

Anyway, a few days into the ashram experience, we'd been doing a lot of dancing. Swirling around, getting our bodies limber and moving in a space where others were doing the same. And then we were shown boxes. Lots of boxes. More than I could count. Each of them contained outfits. Soldiers. Executives. Artists. Children.

You'd change into an outfit, and then wander around the Buddha hall meeting others in costume. And not just in costume. In character. Which is how I came to be Cher for an afternoon. Which might seem like a let down given the way this story started, until you start to consider who we are, how we are, and the nature of the boundaries we hold that define us from not-us...

All of which will make apparent just how important play is in shaping who and what we are. For an insight into that, consider the word *ludicrous*. There's an implication of something larger than life, beyond the norm – all very much to do with things being other than what we're used to. And the root of ludicrous can be found in the Latin ludere - to play. Which is a cue to reflect on some of what led to me prancing around in Cher-drag in the wilds of India.

FORMATIVE INFLUENCES

Childhood was more or less fun. I still think of my relationship with my three sisters as being like The *Waltons*, and the characters in that show had to be resourceful and find ways to get by was reflective of our family experience. We got by, sometimes more than that. Mum and dad had come over from India and worked incredibly hard to support us.

My mother Kamlesh had been a teacher and was on her way to a lecturing role. In England her first job was checking buns passing by on a conveyer belt at Lyons. Later she worked in payroll at Boots, enjoying the teamwork, though also went on to train and work as a teacher here. Between her hours and my dad's long commute, from the age of nine I was pretty much designated female at home.

I'm pretty sure dad Satya has more qualifications and teaching experience than some university departments. Finding the right job was still a stretch, and there was a prolonged period when he worked in London and travelled back to Nottingham where the family have lived for decades. That took its toll. Not just on him, but on dynamics between us all. The fact they and we made it through all this is a testament to their upbringing and character and gives an inkling of what culture and heritage mean in India. Those are very real phenomena which bind people across generations to land and lore.

To uproot your life to another continent and create a new existence allowing you to raise children in is an extraordinary achievement. And the strong sense of connection Kamlesh and Satya had with each other and their own upbringing was about more than the resilience it gave them. My parents are philosophers by nature, and their willingness to explore, build on, and challenge ideas is a defining feature of who they are.

Their outlooks have made a big impact on my own intellectual evolution. As much as anything, philosophy provides tools to think with, knowing that things aren't as simple and wrong. Being able to consider an idea from several angles without either dismissing or embracing, or spiralling into chaos when notions of certainty start to erode, are useful footsteps towards the philosophy – and experience – of spirituality.

FINDING ∧ VOICE

But hey, I was a show-off too. Performing was my thing. A stand-out role as the genie in Aladdin at junior school gave me a boost that was about more than enjoying applause and having fun. (Both of those ticked boxes too, of course.)

None of that surprised dad, who described me as eloquent and confident from an early age.

Early adventures in performance also provided a taste of personal power, though I'd not have thought about it that way at the time. What I did know was pretending to be someone else could be a better experience of being me than I often had on a day-to-day basis.

A lot of this is about boundaries. They define who we are at a given moment. I was a child, a girl, a pupil, a friend, a sister, a daughter. I was of an Indian family and lived in Nottingham. Each of those descriptions marked out an area of who I was in the eyes of others – and myself. And sometimes those labels are inadequate. They can overlap, say. We lived by Melbourne Park, which was a great place to play. Kids loved that, and so mention Melbourne Park and they'd be excited thinking of the fun that could be had.

Adults were different. The park existed between two areas, which made the space ambiguous. At least to estate agents. Thankfully we didn't know any at 10. Anyway, people concerned about property prices wanted to know were we of Wollaton - the posh side of the park - or Aspley... which wasn't.

None of those distinctions meant anything to us as children, only pass-ingly aware of the nuances of this facet of class in Britain. Being brown likewise played a part in how people perceived us as individuals and a family. And with mum employed in working-class and middle-class jobs, then later doing voluntary work, she'd walked between worlds frequently.

One way and another we all do that in different contexts of our lives. And in doing so we develop masks that shape the way we think and act across a range of situations. Part of the fun of drama and singing was intentionally exploring different masks.

I did a pretty deep dive into singing when I lived in London to find ways of dissolving blockages I sensed in my body. For a year I did classes at the Sylvia Young School, which were good but more intended for people who sought fame. I found a tutor called Kate Ramilovik, and studied with her for three years. Getting to know and work with my voice, Kate noted that its deep and tonal resonance made me well suited for use in contexts where getting information across and landing it effectively really matters.

By that point in life, what Kate observed made sense. I had no real desire to win people over for its own sake. Steadily, I'd moved to the realisation that I was on this Earth for a reason and communicating that is how I'd make good use of my vocal talents. All I had to do was work out what my message was...

OUT OF MY BOX

I was brought up in the Hindu faith, without ever really committing to it. The religion itself is beautiful, but at some point I realised I needed to discover what was true or at least useful for myself, rather than rely on preformulated solutions. Hinduism is about compassion, and caring, and love, and has a strong sense of community. All of those qualities have meaning for me, and I've seen them demonstrated time and again in my life – by Hindus, and by people of other faiths or none.

Even when young I had a sense that there was a different way of being, which didn't require beliefs and the stories that go with them. My friends Sarah and Nicola invited me to their Catholic church, where I watched them go into a box to talk to a priest about the things they'd done wrong. Walking home, I noted how mum and dad had told me that if I felt low, or vulnerable, or in need of help, then I could simply breathe slowly and on top of that pray if I wished. And I know those things worked, because I'd used them often when I was the sister-who-coped for my younger sisters when things were difficult.

As an adult, I was learning more for sure. But a lot of it was fuzzy, poorly thought-through, and lacked a practice or focus that would connect intent with reality. There'd be buzzwords a-plenty, and every workshop promised new insights or ancient wisdom, but much of what I encountered was fundamentally empty.

And yet. There were times when I felt connected to something that was older and truer than I was. And at least some of the time it seemed to relate to doing what worked as I began to offer sessions of my own. I was tentative with the massage and meditation and whatever else I was doing at that point, but people were experiencing benefits on a regular basis. Only I knew it was all in a mess. The boxes were all muddled up, and the costumes for yoga chick, energy healer, corporate shaman, and meditation mistress were in the wrong places. Not only that, but none of them fit me properly. At least as Cher's stand-in I had a kickass time knowing just what I was about.

The cosmic turning point happened, as they often do, on a sofa in Ealing, London. But before I sprawled on it, I first had to go to India. I'd visited two times for summers with family as a child. Now, I was returning on a journalistic assignment to interview CEOs and entrepreneurs. Enjoy a few days away in the company of fascinating people and get paid for it. A dream gig. Only, this clearly wasn't my dream any more.

BECOMING MORE LIIKE GOD

After the ashram in 2002, things were definitely opening up. My back wasn't one of them. Not until I went for a massage in Pune. Finding words to describe a transformative experience that involves being twisted and pummelled by a stranger when you're pretty much undressed is tricky. What I do know is this:

Whoever we are, or think we are, isn't just about the mental part of us. Put another way, the experiences that make us the person we are exist at a cellular level. There's much smaller stuff to take into account before you get to cells. A human brain weighs around three pounds, which is pretty much the same as the amount of living bacteria we have. How small are they? Hard to be definitive, but they number in trillions.

Those microbes and cells constitute much of what we are. And they are the building blocks of the larger aspects of us – ones we'd recognise on an X-ray or in the operating theatre scene of a medical drama. The physical activity they are involved in is chemical and electrical in nature. It's affected by what we've eaten, childhood injuries, loving relationships, rewarding work, carbon monoxide, and news media.

That web of influences stretches back in time both genetically – your eye colour and tendency to diabetes, say, and in ways shaped by the experience of ancestors: epigenetics. Hand-me-downs from previous generations can have drastic impact: male descendants of men imprisoned in atrocious conditions in the American Civil War had higher mortality rates than men not of those bloodlines.

A good massage will release some of the material archived in our bodies we no longer need. A neck stiff thanks to work stresses and a poorly designed bag strap. Chest tense because of a failure to breathe fully for too long. Feet sabotaged by evil shoes. That's the stuff you'll know if you've had a massage. And sometimes it's more than that. My Pune massage was a more-than-that massage, squared. Cubed even. It put me back in a better way...eventually.

That massage lit the blue touch paper. By the time I flopped down on the sofa in Ealing, London - seven years later - I was ready to explode, in a kaleidoscopic way that was the most profound spiritual experience of my life.

The notion of being connected to the source, acquired in childhood, got an upgrade. I was hooked right up to the mains. And possibly a bit fried...I got a glimpse of a group of sages in Himalayas. Another me, from another time, was one of them. Not something I ever expected to see, but that's what it was. As well, I seemed to have a direct line to the Vedas, the texts which form the foundation of Hinduism. Which might at least explain why I didn't need to go to temple myself if that material was baked in.

And then I came back. Never mind being knocked for six, I'd been knocked for seven. Maybe more. Thankfully I had a business to occupy me, and make sure I could maintain my lifestyle. Wacky is fine. Wacky and paying the bills is better. And wacky was the word, some of the time. My emotions were in a whirl, and one sister noted that I'd be walking down the street a perfectly sensible woman one minute, laughing hysterically the next.

It took a while to collect my thoughts, compose myself. The idea of being a composition appeals. Music is one of my very favourite things. Getting to be...an aria, a power ballad, a torch song. Yes. They all appealed. Now it was my turn to be Cher. This time unasked, unmasked, as Sunita. Now I could Believe in me.

THE PUPPET SHOW

WHY AYURVEDA

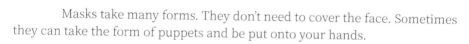

Masks take many forms. They don't need to cover the face. Sometimes they can take the form of puppets and be put onto your hands.

You may know of the performer Rod Hull. He was a ventriloquist, his puppet a large and ill-behaved emu that the entertainer's whole arm went into. It formed a sinewy neck, and a beak that would sneer and peck at people. It's possible you've seen Rod Hull and Emu rampaging on television shows where he'd be a guest and attack the host or an audience member, creating chaos in his wake. Was it Emu doing that, or was it Rod? The answer's not as straightforward as you might imagine, which explains the range of horror stories involving puppets and ventriloquist dummies.

Watching the two of them, it's hard not to get the impression that more than Hull's arm went into his puppet. But at least it was clear that there was a puppet, that a show was going on which – while alarming – was boundaried. It happened on a television screen, where Rod Hull would be just one of a few guests. After a few minutes he'd go off stage and be replaced by a Hollywood actor doing a promotional interview for their new film. They'd be masked too, in a way, there to be amusing and good-looking and make the audience keen to see the movie.

Looked at another way, the actor is a puppet for a billion-dollar corporation whose interests might include oil and gas, publishing, land, and more.

Their face might end up as part of a promotional campaign tied into the film with merchandise available from fast food franchises where kids will delight in fried morsels and a sugary drink. Popped onto the plastic tray taking the meal to a table will be a tie-in item, perhaps a colourful cardboard mask allowing the tiny diner to pretend they're a character played by the actor. Hope for the sake of parents that the character is nothing like Emu.

We are all Emu. Or at any rate sometimes hint at or do a blazing demonstration of our Emu potential. And the way the global economy works at this point encourages such 'give it me right here and right now because I am special and deserve it' behaviour from infancy. Babyfoods that taste sweet even though the flavour on the label suggests savoury condition babies to get that sugary kick early on. Lights and sound and colour in our social and personal environment condition us at every turn and moment. Some of them are useful: red for stop and green to go is an effective way of using technology to make a social contract function effectively for drivers and pedestrians. Others are very much one-sided, or at the very least ambiguous. Places that used to be public and appreciated for their natural beauty or cultural history are splattered with corporate billboards. Advertising shrieks and strobes at us, Emu-ing relentlessly wherever there's a screen to look at. Contemporary manifestations of spirituality too often has an Emu quality: attend a weekend seminar and come back believing that not only do you deserve a Porsche, but the deity of your choice is rooting for you to have it as well.

There's a time and a place for Emu. But it's become the default mode of 21st century interaction online thanks to the way it's cultivated by advertisers and marketeers. The idea that people press buttons in one another has long been a metaphor. Now it's a precision science, sophisticated knowledge of brain chemistry the tool enabling communications to be crafted that will get people excited, agitated, relaxed. Which doesn't mean that we are slaves to whatever machines exist in our homes, our bags, our pockets. But there are moments we are all more or less puppets.

And things are likely to get worse. The red and green traffic lights system has worked for decades. The only light that takes precedence is the blue flashing light on the roof of a police car, or those of other emergency vehicles. There, the purpose is serving the public good. Now, the technology exists to allow some drivers who can pay for the privilege a faster route to their destination through altering the ways traffic flow can be digitally managed. Financial wealth means that someone exceptional for their income gets to do whatever they're travelling to ahead of those exceptional in other ways - like nurses, teachers, and baristas making coffee to keep us alert because it's taking longer to get home.

A NEW CONTEXT FOR AYURVEDA

The changes discussed are ones that affect us all. Where the NHS is going will have a generational impact across UK families. And it's happening against a backdrop where news and social media and the expectations of how we live and work increasingly online are creating their own shifts. Some of them will be good, and that's to be embraced. But much of what's unfolding has ripples that have been coming for decades now. Looking at those requires a brief look at how you can't understand environmental matters without considering the political and economic context in which key choices have been made. Choices are made by people, and those making them are often motivated by self-interest and company mission. The consequences have accelerated crises that are now unavoidably apparent.

Getting through what's happening, and what may be coming, calls for the ability to make better choices for you. And that in turn makes you a resource for family members, friends, and people in other circles of your life. That's the way we get to steer a better path. Not by being diverted by the loudest headline and shiniest new ad. And the best means of doing that, the one I've devoted this existence to, is Ayurveda. Hold that in mind. This material on matters that are political is critical because of what it means for you, your family, your loved ones, and the future of us all. In a storm, you need to be at the eye of it all. And the defining feature of an eye is its ability to see with clarity. Which certainly doesn't mean agreeing with everything written in these pages – but considering the perspectives they present will be valuable.

There's another aspect, too. Ayurveda is a spiritual outlook, and spirituality is often discussed in a way that neuters it. Many who identify as spiritual are so loath to dissent from others who share their sensibilities that they use all-encompassing terms like energy and centred and flow rather than get more specific. General terms can have utility, but such wispiness can also camouflage – mask – an inability to deal with confrontation while assuming communication has happened. Maybe it did, but it's possible there were differences. Exploring them sometimes leads to anxieties about what happens when the nature of those differences is exposed. At which point, passive aggression starts to come out, and once-promising groups fall apart.

Differences are great, but actually engaging with difference is not always straightforward or comfortable in practice. Doing so calls for comprehension and often, consulting several sources of information in addition to those that have been part of our habitual data diet. Which includes learning about things we prefer to keep on a different part of our plate than the bits we like to eat most. All experience is spiritual in some respect, and includes engaging with concepts and truths that may be challenging and require us to change behaviours at a scale bigger and deeper than what we spend our money on.

Running a successful business which has brought me to the attention of transnational corporations has led me both to reinforce my belief in what I'm doing and acknowledge that excessive consumerism is a sickness. Of such paradoxes is a human life made, and it's next-to-impossible to find ways to support yourself in ways that extend your influence without being part of the marketplace. Whether and how you internalise the values of the marketplace is another matter. Acknowledging potential contradictions has sharpened me both as an entrepreneur and as someone whose spiritual practice is active, lived moment by moment.

MEET THE NEW BOSS, REMARKABLY SIMILAR TO THE OLD BOSS

The examples have been at a personal and social level. Self-centred and selfish behaviour has catastrophic consequences on a global scale. Until now, the catastrophe the West has created has largely been confined to countries that get less media attention than celebrity gossip and sports trivia.

So what's happening in those other countries? Africa contains 54 of them. And much of what we hear about Africa is pretty sad. Lots of starving people, economic failure, and social unrest. Charity cases, for reasons that are never adequately explained. Somehow, the people there seem to suck at looking after their countries. The fact Africa contains so many of the world's most vital resources is a useful pointer to that perception: it took a lot of work over many years to create the racist and erroneous picture presented of the world's second biggest continent. It got that way by intent. John Perkins blew the whistle on the role he played in his contribution, when he was employed to undermine African economies for the benefit of American corporations, in the book *Confessions of an Economic Hit-man*.

In his job as the Chief Economist of a big consultancy firm Perkins convinced not just governments but the World Bank and International Monetary Fund that nations in Africa and elsewhere would benefit from infrastructure investment. The packages were presented in ways that made them look unmissable, but were engineered to fail. That failure meant the country owed even more to America, meaning corporations with government and CIA backing get to determine the fate of that nation. Methods used include assassination. Oil companies in particular benefit from a system that leaves workers are underpaid with no rights.

Before American involvement in Africa there was the British Empire. From the British, America learned that it was better not to be directly involved with the countries being exploited: it takes a lot of boots on the ground to do that. And now the Americans have been usurped in turn, by China. That opportunity was presented by the shift from the 20th century's oil economy to the 21st where, as the saying goes, 'data is the new oil'. And anything to do with digital data is ultimately reliant on rare earth minerals used in phones and computers – those minerals can be found in abundance in Africa.

Countries in Africa know to be wary of American promises. China knows that. Instead of offering unmeetable deals for unrepayable investment, China has instead gone ahead and got on with and delivered the infrastructure projects that African nations sought the money for. In return, it's the Chinese that now control much of the world's supply of those rare earth minerals. And they're getting active in agriculture in Africa too, at a point when food supplies are going to be an increasingly contentious issue because the world faces unparalleled instances of systemic environmental collapse thanks to commitment to uncontrolled growth for the last century.

LESS EMU, MORE CHER

As an achievement, all this plunder and domination is a startling achievement in its scale and devastation – environmentally, socially, psychically. Emu has gone around the world bossing people about and eating their food, and more of them than we'd like to think have become Emu to bully others and steal what they have. The word for this is, of course, Emulation.

Some of the lookalikes are corporate bosses, who are easy to spot, and include many amazing people as I know from my journalistic days. Others can pop up in the form of online influencers, social enterprises, Instagram-friendly yoginis. Some are well-intentioned but lack method. Others have intent, but not the sort you'd want to be caught up in. What the world needs now is Cher, sweet Cher, to get people singing the song of Ayurveda.

WHY AYURVEDA, WHY NOW?

At the heart of Ayurveda are a set of principles and practice that support a balanced life. They were developed over centuries in India, and embody many generations of people who took the approach on board without it being a fad, a cult, or someone's power trip. Ayurveda was simply a way to approach living that you knew worked because that's what it had done for your great grandparents, your grandparents, and your parents.

In the morning, you'd eat at a time that made sense for your body. Other family members might eat as you did, or have something different. The vision of a full English or a line of American-style cereals with everyone having a favourite based on food colouring didn't exist.

Also in the morning, and at other times of the day, you might want to enjoy music. Ayurveda would have a suggestion for the kind of playing that would suit the energy of the moment. Maybe some body yoga would form part of the way you woke and welcomed the world. And meditation then or at some other point would likely be part of how you kept your balance as one day turned into another. None of this was set in stone. Eating because your type - dosha is the term used - wasn't simply about your body type – it was also a way of understanding temperament, and how stresses might be expressed for you. You might have skin problems while your brother experiences bowel issues, but be fundamentally similar in other respects. And your dosha itself wasn't a fixed thing. There were three, and you could be mostly one, but have touches of the others in different contexts at different times.

That fluidity exists in regard to nutrition, as well. Eating well is important, but food is neither a status symbol or succour. What you eat matters, and is matter, and is energy too in Ayurvedic understanding. So why would you want to eat something that will cause you harm? Why make food the solution for a problem that actually exists in your relationship with another person? How will developing an ulcer make it more possible to have the talk you've been dreading? Maybe a massage using oils made from particular plants grown on the same farm for a century now would relieve whatever tension you're holding, and allow you both to meet up and have the discussion that will clear the air.

Already from this you'll be getting a sense of how Ayurveda is a non-dogmatic system that's not about being right but instead offers practical time-tested ways to do things which will be beneficial. If you get ill there's going to be someone who can help you, but for the most part knowledge within your own family will keep you pretty much on track thanks to centuries of examples of how Ayurveda simply works. And because the dosha-based approach could be applied in new contexts as well as ones people were familiar with, they could make an informed attempt to deal with something new, that nobody in their lineage had come across.

Did Ayurveda always work? No. Does anything always work? No. And if it failed to be useful, was the failure one of Ayurveda? Or an example of applying principles in a context where they don't fit? Or of not noticing a salient detail? All of these are less to do with Ayurveda, than of humans being human. Ayurveda only exists through the humans who practice it. And the more we practice, the more we learn. Ayurveda provides templates and guidelines, rather than being an all-encompassing instruction manual. People in India developed gout, went crazy in scary ways, had menopause difficulties and bad hair days as humans have for millennia. They just had a very cool toolkit for coping. They had Ayurveda.

You'll notice in all of this there's no mention of the word medicine. Essentially, in Ayurveda, everything is medicine. If you're eating well in accord with your dosha and season, then there's no need to have anything else in your system than the food you've already chosen. And some of the same ingredients will be there in a preparation, along with some others if needed. Herbs can be used in different ways, and different parts of one plant could be used to deal with a range of conditions.

All of this points to Ayurveda being an evolving system based on an essentially scientific approach. There's a body of knowledge to refer to, and using that core information it's possible to develop new solutions in line with a previously unencountered situation. The Sanskrit word Ayuh means life, or vitality, or longevity, and Vedah means knowledge, or science. Pretty much then, it's a science of life. And it's one you don't have to be approved to study by the British Medical Association, but learn from childhood as a member of a community where it's been woven into life for centuries...millennia in fact. Ayurveda has existed certainly since 1500BC, and potentially for longer.

LEARNED HELPLESSNESS

The idea that you need to have your health needs attended to by medical professionals rather than being responsible for your own wellbeing is problematic. There's an implicit underpinning that a doctor can fix what's broken, rather than you and those around you taking responsibility for keeping you out of hospital in the first place.

Ivan Illich offered an examination of the failings of that system and culture in his book Medical *Nemesis*. He noted that faith in experts reduces the willingness and competence people have in dealing with their own health issues. And the repercusions are terrifying.

You may or may not know what *iatrogenesis* means. You have very likely come across its consequences. The word describes the inadvertent results of what happens as a result of treatment in a medical system designed to heal but which is estimated to be the 5th largest cause of death in the world. That's the conclusion of an article providing a good overview of the subject by RF Peer and N. Shabir Peer RF, *Iatrogenesis: A review on nature, extent, and distribution of healthcare hazards*. J Family Med Prim Care 2018;7:309-14

Put another way, the doctors and hospitals we trust to heal us constitute one of the world's principle causes of our premature demise. Sometimes the issue is adverse drug reactions. It can be poor communication within complicated bureaucracies. Another category is unsafe practices such as botched injections – botched blood transfusions were responsible for between 5% and 15% of HIV infections according to a 2008 WHO report.

Drugs don't have to be badly prescribed to be dangerous. Purdue Pharma, manufacturers of Oxycontin, bribed doctors and distributors to push an addictive opioid that killed over half a million Americans. In the process they made as much as $13 billion, and the Sackler family who headed the company used some of that wealth to create a reputation as philanthropists.

It's not even possible to show a need for Oxycontin that grows in line with rising levels of physical or emotional suffering between 1999 and 2009 when use of the drug was escalating. The key difference was the marketing for the product itself, accompanied by misleading claims about its safety and widespread use of incentives for doctors to prescribe the drug.

When the system is sick, the patient becomes irrelevant. You only have to look at what happened to pop icon Britney Spears. The child star turned global phenomenon was under the conservatorship of her father owing to her mental health problems. Britney was forced to use a contraceptive device against her wishes, and use the psychiatric drug Lithium, while performing shows that have bankrolled not just her father but the legal and medical professionals involved in looking after her best interests.

It's difficult not to read the details of a case like Britney's and see there's something deeply wrong happening in the world. There is. And in many ways we are all its victims. If Cher is one heroine who shows the way forward, let Britney be an icon for those of us determined to create a viable future on our own terms.

I AM BRITNEY (AND SO ARE YOU)

It doesn't have to be this way.

In the film Spartacus, gladiator Kirk Douglas leads a revolt. The Roman authorities are determined to find their man. He stands alongside his fellow rebels, and the Romans ask which of them is Spartacus. Before he can state his identity, one of those standing by him claims to be Spartacus. Then another, and another, until there's no way the powers-that-be can distinguish who is who any more. They're all trouble-makers.

It's worth thinking about, and putting together with Britney's story. You can claim your own wellbeing. Learn to be a champion for those matters of health you can influence using the timeless techniques and knowledge of Ayurveda.

Do it for you.

Do it for your family.

Do it for your friends.

Do it for your community.

Do it for the future.

And do it in the name and spirit of Britney, or whoever else stands for you as representing a loving rebel spirit determined to do what's right to challenge a system that's lost its way and become self-interested.

At the moment we're experiencing a world where old certainties are withering. They won't be replaced by anything constructive and generative unless we do it ourselves, person by person. We don't have to know everything or get it all right. Neither do those who benefit from the way things are run currently, and which creates human misery, animal exploitation, and environmental devastation on a global scale.

We need a blueprint for a better life. Ayurveda certainly doesn't have all the answers, and was never intended to. What it does do is provide a template for living differently that allows us to ask questions together and take responsibility for ourselves and those around us, rather than rely on those who demonstrably do not have our interests at heart.

What's good about now we can keep. And those are questions we can ask too. The planet cannot sustain the way we're living at the moment, and the versions of the future being presented don't look rosy for the great majority of us. We need to look after ourselves as that future emerges, and Ayurveda is a loving way forward into the years ahead.

OUT OF WHACK

NUTRITION

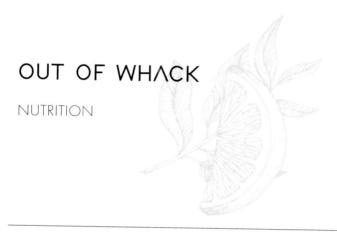

If Ayurveda equips us with ways to notice and act about the ways we're balanced, and what to do about when we notice we're out of equilibrium. That concept is an interesting one, suggesting as it does that there's a best or at least better version of ourselves that we have at least some awareness of, and can compare our day-to-day condition to. Which is pretty useful. Recognising you're having a bad hair day allows you to choose an appropriate shampoo...bad hair can be metaphorical and ditto choice of product.

Unfortunately, when it comes to choice of product, we've been conned for decades. Many businesses are intent on selling us more of what they believe we want, whether or not we need it. And the psychology of advertising is essentially about tricking people into believing they have either specific inadequacies particular products can fix, or that they're generally worthless but that there is at least some respite. It could be a BMW, if you have that kind of income. For many more, it's a quick hit of sugars and fats contained in a brightly coloured package (mass market) or something classier made in smaller numbers. Either way, you stuff it down your gullet and after the initial buzz guilt often follows.

You could look at guilt as a chance for course-correction, but again that's been turned against us thanks to psychologists and media. Church too, for those who've had a bad version of it. The weight loss industry is enormous, making gross amounts of money from people who the businesses involved know will be back soon, whether attending classes, or buying low-calorie prepared meals and misery-making books.

BACK ON TRACK

It's all a long way from what the ancient writer Charaka described millennia ago:

"The life of all things is food and the entire world seeks food."

Hmm. At that point not far from a PowerPoint slide in a marketing meeting for a conglomerate. Charaka goes on:

"Complexion, clarity, good voice, long life, understanding, happiness, satisfaction, growth, strength and intelligence are all established in food."

By now, board members would be curious and potentially excited at the revenue streams about to open up with this bold new approach to delivering calories. But that wasn't what Charaka had in mind.

Ayurveda recognises people are equipped with the makings of wisdom and self-control and capacity to learn that allow them to make choices about what they consume so their meals and drinks actively nourish them. (Ponder the differences between **nourish** and **consume** while we're on the subject.)

There's a Sanskrit word which sums all this up, and that word is **swasthavritta**. Sanskrit is a poetic language that uses words in nuanced ways so that their meanings are layered. Tooth and egg and Brahmin, for instance, are united by concepts of being twice-born in the word **dvija**. Lose a tooth and another pops up in its place. A bird is conceived first by its parents, and then emerges from an egg. Similarly, a Brahmin – a priest whose responsibilities may include transmitting teachings about Ayurvedic nutrition - experiences a kind of rebirth through initiation.

Swasthavritta similarly has quite a few ideas in all those letters, though bear in mind the original text looks very different.

Swastha – innate, natural, inherent, of the self.
Sta – to stand, and to live well.
Av – to protect, and do good.
Vritta – using the senses correctly, better choices, compassion for self.

Put them together and you end up with a word that could be put as "An individual's stand to nurture and protect life." In there, you've got notions of harmony and of balance and health. Implicit too are concepts of positivity and connection. Positivity in this sense isn't about hoping for the best and sending fuzzy vibes. Do those by all means, but back them up by making decisions and living with their consequences. This isn't the outlook of a passive consumer. Standing and protecting life involves relation with community and environment. It's the stance of someone who finds ways to be actively involved in the world.

That perspective follows when you appreciate the extent to which eating in line with ingredients and spices suited to your constitution can prevent many illnesses appearing in the first place. The preventative outlook is a healthier and happier way to live than one based on cures reliant on pharmaceuticals (whether in medicine, or food), the machinations of the diet industry, or various forms of therapy. Which doesn't mean that all can have a role to play for some people some of the time. But it's not hard to see that a culture which presents the obese with a menu of options including surgical removal of fat, or clamping their jaws so food can only be ingested through a straw, is seriously messed-up. Then take a look at how people got that way, and meditate on feeders: women (typically) who eat grotesque amounts of food in return for payment by men (mostly) who derive sexual satisfaction from those who achieve life-threatening weight.

BETTER QUESTIONS PRODUCE BETTER ANSWERS

Rather than assuming a person is somehow broken and needs assistance from a professional claiming expertise, starting with your own situation and being with that will often provide the information needed to create change for the better. With some of the information and ways of thinking Ayurveda provides, you've got a diagnostic tool allowing you to draw useful conclusions and act on them.

Ask yourself a question like "Why am I not digesting properly?" and you're primed to reflect on recent eating habits (or maybe ones stretching further back) in light of a key organising principle which needs a couple more words to be introduced. Those words are ojas and agni. And there's a whole cosmology packed away in their eight letters and four syllables. Their remit includes but is not limited to food. Think of them as directing and coordinating essence and quality, particularly at a physical level – which naturally involves what we eat and drink.

OJAS is concerned with...	**AGNI incorporates...**
Spiritual growth	Digestive fire
Vigour, energy for body/mind	Stomach, considered akin to an engine
Strength, endurance	Digestion, a fundamental process in...
Health, vitality levels	Assimilation, transformation

The relationship of agni and ojas can affect all aspects of how our bodies function, specifically with what's called dhatus, otherwise known as the seven tissues. Please don't feel you need to know all these names by the way – what matters more is having a sense for the way Ayurveda has long had an appreciation for how systems interact. And doing so requires a way to think about the aspects of that system. In this case, they are:

Rasa – lymph/plasma
Rakta – blood
Mamsa – muscle
Medas – fat
Asthi – bone
Majja – marrow/nerve
Shukra – reproductive organs

What that means is problems showing up in any of those seven tissues can be considered as manifestations of ojas and agni. It may help to look at how another system with two intertwining factors can affect a whole range of subsidiary phenomena.

IT'S YOUR TURN

Consider the esoteric duo Money and Time in the context of food as you consider these more-serious-than-they-look questions. And be honest. Nobody's looking at your answers waiting to judge them.

How much were you spending on take-out coffee to make your job doable before lockdown? What are you doing with that money now?

Would you rather devote a day to making a meal for family and friends or spend the day doing work you love and go to a special restaurant with them?

How important is convenience where choosing food is concerned?

If you were going to grow your own vegetables, how would you consider the investment in time to acquire the skills and maintain the soil? What financial sacrifice might that represent and how would you justify it if you feel the need to?

When you consider the choices others make about food, to what extent are you judging them by beliefs about money and time that might not apply to their lives?

That ability to think about the interplay of different influences in your life and life at large makes Ayurveda not so much a path with answers but a prompt for investigating what can work for you, making use of a body of knowledge but not being restricted to it.

Anyway, those are the kind of things people are getting at when they talk about systems and the tangled forces at work in them. Ayurveda couldn't be more everyday, in other words. It only initially sounds otherwise because of its long history, the unfamiliar words, and it being part of something people call spiritual.

Look at the seven dhatus through the filters of agni and ojas and the questions popping up can work like the ones about money and time that already inform your thinking. 'How come I have an allergy to apples now it's winter but I never had in the summer?'. The effect is like looking through a microscope or even a kaleidoscope - maybe a bit confusing initially but soon enough something comes into view that might shed light.

It may turn out the summer apples are in season, and local. The winter ones may have come from another country, and been treated with a preservative in a warehouse (whether or not they need one) that's problematic for you. Within the scope of what that lens presents, all kinds of ideas can pop up. Some of them resemble what have become fads in a western context – paleo and dairy-free are two examples. Rather than being a One True Way as new dietary approaches are sometimes presented, in Ayurvedic terms they clearly present a viable solution that will be right for some people, some of the time.

NO, DOSHAS HAVEN'T BEEN MENTIONED SO FAR

This far into a book on Ayurveda you'd expect to read about **doshas**, which are the nugget that most people with a passing acquaintance or more will be aware of beyond what's in the public consciousness such as meditation and massage. We'll get to them in due course. Shorthand version is they are descriptions of how we are likely to think, feel, and respond based on physiology and temperament.

The danger in presenting a concept you have prior familiarity with is that it reduces the prospect of learning something new by filing it as 'stuff I understand'. In this case, the ideas already discussed lay the ground for a better understanding of doshas – and more. That in mind, consider the following:

Don't mistake the fact that doshas or any other set of categories usefully describing how someone is at a given moment in time for a label which describes them reliably long term. That's a shortcut to disappointment when you discover the person you tagged as being one kind of person shows there's more to them. And you might have spotted that if you'd been flexible and perceptive enough to read the signs rather than telling yourself you know the score. You don't, and never will. The belief that a placeholder which worked on one or more given occasions allows you to be upset and let down when the person you applied them to behaves differently is a problem for you, and not them.

WE ARE WHAT WE EAT

We are spiritual beings living in a world of matter. Sustaining ourselves as well as we can requires us to eat. And there are ways we can do that which as well as supporting our physical health can also benefit our mental and emotional state. And as with a lot of Ayurveda, you can recognise the core truth of that in your own experience.

If you're feeling lethargic, and sinking into old habits and unhelpful thoughts, which is it more likely that you've been eating? Fresh fruit and vegetables served with whole grains? Or white sliced bread, processed foods, and leftovers from who knows how far back?

Odds are you've answered the second. Which are all associated with *tamasic* ways of thinking, which is all about stuckness. *Tamas* is about inertia.

All that fresh food meanwhile is sattvic in nature, which encourages our higher qualities: openness, curiosity, kindness, and love. *Sattva* is about purity.

Warm and stimulating foods such as good quality meat, eggs, chickpeas, and red lentils encourage *rajasic* qualities - movement and passion...too much can lead to frustration and anger. Rajas is about activity.

AS ABOVE, SO BELOW

We've got down to the matter of what's on your plate finally. And in looking at it, we're seeing how one product of creation on this planet we share – animals and plants – sustains another...humankind. Which underlines that our choices matter. They affect not just us, but ripple out to the social sphere. Low blood sugar has been accepted as a contributing factor in murder cases. What children do or don't eat at the start of day impacts their ability to learn. Oh, and get things wrong with the way we approach other inhabitants of Earth, whatever their species, and the planet will be fine. It can manage without us.

Those choices are there every day in the food we select. And in making those choices we side with one or another Hindu deity. Each of them lines up with the tamasic, sattvic, and rajasic foods mentioned above...

Brahma, the Creator - rajas
Vishnu, the Preserver - sattva
Shiva, the Destroyer – tamas

Next time you go to your fridge, think about that. Which deity do you want to dine with?

IT'S YOUR TURN

Already you've come across a lot of information in this chapter. It's fine. You don't need to take it all on board just like that.

Consider your own relationship with nutrition in the light of the concepts already presented. Test them in your experience rather than taking it for granted that this or any other book knows you better than you do.

When you've made some progress on that front, check out the ideas that follow. Keep a food diary, and as you keep it bear these pointers in mind.

- Investigate doshas as if you're doing it from scratch, regardless of how familiar you are with using them.
- Explore the natural qualities of foods. Those innate characteristics are termed gunas.
- Think through how those qualities get altered. What factors go into that? Is ingredient freshness an issue? Season perhaps?
- Food combination: how does it work for you when you mix food types? What have you learned to avoid, and what does that suggest? What works great together?
- Mathra is about quantity of food. How much is right for you to consume, bearing in mind the suggestion that you should feel hungry a couple of times daily?
- The remit of desha is where food is grown, prepared, and consumed.
- The when of food is important, whether seasonal – ruthu – or within a day – kala.
- What is the effect of chemicals in your diet? Preservatives, colouring, artificial flavourings, and other additives.

INTRODUCING MIRANDA BOSCAWEN

I'm fortunate to have met people in the UK who adopt Ayurveda in more truthful ways than some I've known in India and been brought up with it. Sometimes it's about personality. And need makes a real difference too.

Miranda Boscawen was diagnosed with cancer close to two decades ago. Technically it's a condition she still has, and her doctors comment on how remarkable Miranda's health is – especially since she's never had chemo treatment or radiation. She credits that vibrancy in large part to a fundamental change in diet that she learned from Ayurveda. Miranda is a great example of the principle that teachers learn from those they taught, which is why I thought I'd turn to her to ask for some of the specifics she's acquired in changing the way she eats.

Above all else, bear this in mind:

Eating a variety of fresh, organic, seasonal, foods will provide the best nutritional profile.

More detailed suggestions in line with that overall proposition:

1.   BUY FRESH

People often think they can't afford fresh food, but when bought regularly then it's possible to plan meals rather than relying on impulse buys. And because plans never go to plan, you also get the random joy of making soups with that leftover carrot, courgette stub, and cabbage remnants. Tasty, especially with some herbs and spices in stock. And as well as being healthier, often a way to save money compared to anything packaged or processed. Just bear in mind that the fresher the food the higher the nutritional value is likely to be. The longer the food hangs around the more nutritional value will be lost.

2.   BUY ORGANIC

Organic or even better biodynamic farming https://www.biodynamic.org.uk/ considers how the animal and/or land is cared for. Research demonstrates significant nutritional differences between foods produced organically and non-organically. While side by side on a supermarket shelf organic produce might look more expensive, realise you are buying foods with higher nutritional value. Cows are designed to move around eating grasses not stand inside eating corn, so pay extra for that exercise routine!

It's data-time!

Higher antioxidant levels were found in organic crops along with lower concentrations of pesticides. [1]

Organic milk and meat contain around 50% more beneficial anti-inflammatory omega-3 fatty acids than non-organic.[2]

This also applies to organic dairy like butter, cream, cheese and yoghurt. Many people in western countries have too much too much pro-inflammatory omega-6 fatty acids in their diet, often from high intake of vegetable oils in processed foods. Fats in meat from grain fed cows are high in omega 6.

Other health benefits can be demonstrated by a recent investigation into the effect of organic milk consumption on eczema in children younger than 2 years...eczema was significantly reduced in children from families consuming organic rather than non-organic milk.[3]

3.   BUY SEASONAL

Buying seasonally helps ensure we eat a wider range of foods. The importance of seasonal eating is best demonstrated in deer. Eating foods not in season can kill a deer and this is something we too should take note of. Out of season foods can be harder to digest. Good gut health is supported by eating seasonally. Ayurveda has long understood the importance of seasonal changes.

4.   BUY THE RAINBOW

Each different coloured food provides different benefits. Eating as many colours as possible will ensure you receive plentiful phytonutrients helping to prevent disease. Think beta-carotene in carrots, Lycopene in tomatoes, sulforaphane in spinach, allicin in onions and flavonoids in blueberries.

---

1 https://www.cambridge.org/core/journals/british-journal-of-nutrition/article/higher-antioxidant-and-lower-cadmium-concentrations-and-lower-incidence-of-pesticide-residues-in-organically-grown-crops-a-systematic-literature-review-and-metaanalyses/33F09637EAE6C4ED119E0C4BFFE2D5B1#

2 https://www.cambridge.org/core/journals/british-journal-of-nutrition/article/higher-pufa-and-n3-pufa-conjugated-linoleic-acid-tocopherol-and-iron-but-lower-iodine-and-selenium-concentrations-in-organic-milk-a-systematic-literature-review-and-meta-and-redundancy-analyses/A7587A524F4235D8E98423E1F73B6C05

3 https://www.cambridge.org/core/journals/british-journal-of-nutrition/article/composition-differences-between-organic-and-conventional-meat-a-systematic-literature-review-and-metaanalysis/B333BC0DD4B-23193DDFA2273649AE0EE

OUT OF WHACK - NUTRITION   49

5.   BUY LOCAL

Wherever you live, eat the food that is in season there. There are so many benefits to buying locally, and from a nutritional standpoint, buying locally makes it easier to eat fresher, seasonal foods. You can also build a relationship with your local farms and find those that limit using pesticides and preservatives. Even organic foods such as apples when bought in supermarkets are often waxed to preserve them when they are travelling from the other side of the world. Why buy apples from New Zealand when British apples are in season? Many farms offer weekly box deliveries. Find a food box scheme near you https://www.foodboxes.org/

6.   STORAGE

a)   Avoid frozen as much as possible. Fruits and vegetables start to deteriorate as soon as they are picked. Foods bought frozen can be an alternative to fresh food where the produce is picked when ripe and flash frozen straight away to preserve the nutrients. If you are freezing at home don't wait to freeze produce as there will be a loss of nutrients as well as colour and flavour. Some foods are blanched before freezing to prevent loss of colour. If blanching food at home to freeze, the produce should be plunged into cold water immediately afterwards to prevent it from cooking further. To preserve the nutrients don't overcook the vegetables before freezing. Blanching vegetables such as broccoli before freezing will help prevent it turning to mush when you want to use it. Soft fruits such as raspberries or blackberries are best laid out on a tray after picking and part frozen until firm before being bagged or boxed. This will help preserve their form.

b)   Buy or preserve food in glass jars if you can't shop regularly. Preserve as soon after picking or buying as possible. All sorts of foods can be kept in this way; fruits and vegetables as well as eggs, meats and fish. The exact method depends on the food. There are lots of books available to get you started with preserving food.

c)   Most tins for food are today lined with BPA (bisphenol A) plastic. This stops the metal tin corroding...and allows the BPA to migrate from the lining into the food. And you. BPA (or BPS or BPF) is thought to mimic the structure and function of estrogen, binding to estrogen receptors and other hormone receptors having an effect on cell growth and repair and reproduction.

7.   READ THE INGREDIENTS

Ultra-processed foods should be avoided altogether. They are usually highly refined, high in artificial ingredients, chemically altered sugars, and other refined carbs as well as salts and bad fats. Don't be drawn in by names of fake farms (actually brand names), pretty pictures and marketing spiel on a packet.

Avoid foods with ingredients that can't be grown in a garden or reared on a farm! Be wary of anything that says low sugar or low fat – these are often far worse than eating natural fats and unrefined sugars. Especially avoid artificial sweeteners such as aspartame.
Other ingredients to watch out for include refined sugar syrups and margarine (even flies don't like it!).

With the drive to eat vegan a lot more ready-made foods and bakery items now use margarine in place of butter. Steer clear of anything hydrogenated, such as partially hydrogenated oils. Often healthy-looking foods such as yoghurts and smoothies are loaded with added sugars so read that label!

8.   ENJOY LEARNING NEW RECIPES AND TECHNIQUES

Buy as much as you can in fresh ingredient form to cook from scratch. If your cooking skills aren't sophisticated stretch with home-made muffins. They're great for breakfasts and lunch boxes while shop bought versions tend to be loaded with refined sugars, artificial sweeteners, and preservatives. There are some great Muffin recipes here https://www.naturedoc.co.uk/?s=muffins

If you take to baking muffins, consider moving onto bread. If you're ready for that step, there are plenty of sources out there. And start by checking out good commercial breads. Traditional bakers are making a comeback but if you can't find one near you Waitrose sell Bertinet Bakery Bread as whole loaves or sliced made using traditional methods. https://bertinetbakery.com/

Paying more for your bread is really worth it. Bread should not have hydrogenated oils in it or a long list of ingredients. Watch for high sugar levels. Sourdough can be made simply with flour, water & sea salt. If you won't eat a whole loaf, slice and put it in the freezer. Oxford based Modern Baker is on a mission to make "healthy baking available to everyone" Baked by science you can now buy their bread on Amazon! https://www.modernbaker.com/

9.   HERBS, AND WHERE TO FIND THEM

There's centuries of lore within Ayurveda about the benefits of herbs of various kinds, many of which can be used in making meals. You'll probably know about the incredible digestive benefits of ginger already: it's also an antioxidant and anti-inflammatory among other things. Its relative turmeric has similar advantages, and is good for easing tension. You may not know all of these herbs, which have considerable research evidence...

Ashwagandha is a stress-reliever. Great for relaxing, as is *tulsi* (Holy basil).

Bacopa is good for boosting the brain. Calms the mind and aids memory.

Triphala is a formula of three plants effective as a laxative and helps you absorb nutrients.

Neem has effect on autcommimmune disorders and is good for plaque and skin conditions.

Shatavari is great for issues involving the reproductive system for women, useful for menstrual problems and menopause. Men too experience benefits.

The obvious question is the extent to which using Indian herbs is problematic for those in the UK given transport issues means by the time we get them here they're not fresh. They're also, of course, not local. A brilliant researcher called Anne McIntyre has looked into this extensively, and discovered analogs for those Indian plants which grow in the British Isles. Check out what she's doing over at annemcintrye.com

Regarding turmeric and other herbs in prepared forms, selecting a quality company with commitment to Ayurveda will make all the difference. High street names will use smoke and mirrors to convince you theirs is just as good, but for Indian herbs of therapeutic standard it's worth checking out the range at essentialayurveda.co.uk – in particular look at their Chyawanprash, a formulation using 25 herbs and spices combined with the amla fruit. Its benefits around circulation, immune system, rejuvenation and more are well attested.

There's an old saying that an army marches on its belly. It's true for families, couples, individuals even. What we nourish ourselves with is one of the biggest parts of who we are and what we become. Making better choices can be life-transforming, as it has been for Miranda Boscawen. You can learn more about Miranda, and have sessions with her in the Oxford area, here: http://avitallife.co.uk/

One of the recipes that's a classic in Ayurveda for its restorative qualities is *kitchari*, one of those dishes that tastes so good you can't believe it's healthy. Kitchari is traditionally made from either yellow lentils or split peas, basmati rice, a mixture of digestive spices, and ghee. The theory behind this dish's efficacy has a lot to do with the concept of food combining. A mono-nutrient fast gives our digestive systems a much-needed break from dealing with a mess of different foods in every meal. The dal and rice is cooked until just short of mush, making it easier to absorb. The spice mix fires up our belly, and the ghee (or coconut oil) helps lube up your tubing and allows fat-soluble nutrients to assimilate. This recipe comes from Julie Dent, a long-time client and now friend whose Ayurvedic spa retreat The Clover Mill is a joy. www.theclovermill.com

Prep time 10 minutes

Cook time 45 minutes

Servings 4

Ingredients:

- 1 cup dried yellow split peas or lentils
- 1 cup basmati rice
- 3 tablespoons ghee or coconut oil
- 1 tablespoon grated fresh ginger
- 2 teaspoons ground cumin
- 1 teaspoon ground coriander
- 1 teaspoon fennel seeds
- 1 teaspoon ground fenugreek
- 1 teaspoon ground turmeric
- 1 teaspoon sea salt

- 5 cups vegetable stock or water
- 2 cups of fresh green veg finely chopped into an almost rice-like texture
- 1/4 cup coriander
- Plain full-fat Greek yoghurt for serving (optional)

Instructions:

1. Rinse the yellow split peas or lentils and rice in a fine mesh colander under cold water until the water runs clear.
2. In a large-lidded saucepan over medium-high heat, heat the coconut oil or ghee. Add the ginger and cook, stirring, for 30 seconds. Add the cumin, coriander, fennel seeds, fenugreek, and turmeric. Cook for another 30 seconds, until fragrant.
3. Add the split peas or lentils and rice and stir to coat in the spices. Add the salt and pour in the water or vegetable stock. Bring to a boil, cover, and reduce the heat to medium/low. Simmer for 35-45 minutes, stirring occasionally, until the peas/lentils are tender but not mushy and most of the liquid has been absorbed. (You may need to add more water if the mixture becomes to dry or begins to stick to the bottom of the pan).
4. Stir in the green veg. Cover and cook for another 4-5 minutes, then remove from the heat and leave to stand for 5 minutes. Serve warm, scattered with coriander and plain yoghurt if desired.

LOOKING BΛCK TO LOOK FORWΛRD

HERBAL REMEDIES

On my father's side, my great grandfather Ram Chandara Passi was a landowner and money lender with a reputation for philanthropy that benefited the community. He wasn't an educated man but had an appreciation that modest wealth had its source in those around him and felt a responsibility to use it to nurture the community and not just his family.

My grandfather Sardari Lal Passi was the first person in the village of Sabhra to receive a college education, from a college in Lahore. He embraced his father's wisdom about community and added to that learning which made him a good listener as well as an impressive orator.

Grandad's connection to land was innate. He knew where he was from, and that his relationship with that place mattered. Animals were part of that bond. Father said the way his dog barked was a clear indication of whether a visitor's intent was good or otherwise. Grandad also had a horse and kept chickens. And when he began his Ayurvedic practice he worked with local farmers to cultivate the herbs and plants that would be used in his medicines.

There's a fundamental distinction between that kind of outlook and the one that's typically seen in the western approach to pharmaceutical research. Interest might be expressed in plants, but primarily for the molecules that are understood to be what makes something useful happen in a specific health context.

The concept that people and land and plants and animals co-exist is alien to many. But it's only recently even in western history that such has been the case. Workers tempted by regular employment and homes were lured to towns and cities across Britain. Over time, their family networks weakened. Emphasis on shift work took away time that would have been spent in communal activities and sharing knowledge and skills.

People had money to spend on new distractions such as cinema, cars, and foreign holidays – all with a place in their lives, but also leading to an erasure of expertise and understanding over time. It's essentially a less brutal version of what indigenous populations in America, Canada, and Australia among other places – India included – since encountering the west.

Ayurveda is my tradition, my heritage. It's in my blood. Descendants of the farmers who grew herbs and plants for my grandfather now grow them for my Tri-Dosha products. That continuity is important to me. In a different way to what was possible for my grandfather, I am now finding ways to continue that lineage in a 21st century context.

One advantage I have is access to wider sources of information, both through books and digital media, and through the people and places I've experienced in my travels. Sometimes it's useful to look outside your own culture to see how others are working in parallel ways. If Ayurveda has truth, others will have found a version of it with descriptions matching a worldview shaped by their own mythologies.

GLIMPSES OF OTHER WAYS

Lenny Darnell is an American who lived with an Amazonian tribe – not studying them as an anthropologist, but one of the gang, something he did alongside being a business consultant and excellent pianist. One of the things that took Lenny's interest was how people got knowledge of the rainforest they lived in.

Lenny spoke with a shaman and asked how they knew what plants would benefit someone with a sickness. He asked in part to discover if that knowledge was handed down, which would suggest over several generations information would dwindle because of the human tendency to forget. Instead the shaman told Lenny — as if it was the most straightforward thing in the world — that when he wanted that kind of knowledge he would ask the forest. It was an answer that perplexed Lenny. Asking the forest? What does that even mean?

For a while Lenny sat with his confusion. Some thinking, and a decidedly 21st century mobile phone call to a notably smart mentor - NLP co-creator Richard Bandler - led him to ask *where* in the forest the shaman asked his question. And the shaman told Lenny about the rock he stood on, in front of a waterfall, where he'd direct his question to the waters he faced.

At the time, Lenny was suffering from a skin condition. He went with the shaman to the waterfall and stood on the rock as instructed. Then supposed he could communicate as instructed, making a vivid mental picture of his skin condition. Almost instantly — *wham* —Lenny had a detailed image of a plant in his head where none had been before. He described its particulars to the shaman, who was able to find one and use it in a preparation which successfully treated what was happening with Lenny's skin.

It's easy to find parallels with Ayurveda there. A broad, deep, and expanding lore dating back millennia which many have some knowledge of, and where a group of practitioners build on that tradition as they encounter new conditions, and different plants. The Hindu concept of devas is pertinent here: think of them as spirits, tens of millions or even more in number, involved with life in all its forms – including plants.

Go back to an early Ayurvedic practice outlined in the collection of texts known as *Caraka Samhita*, and in gathering herbs for healing a practitioner is advised to offer the plant they found a floral offering – *archana* – to honour its deva. Next day, return to ask for its consent. This would sometimes be done with the aid of a text written on a preserved palm leaf, commencing with a *Mangala Charana*, an address to the deities and devas involved, followed by the specifics of why the plant is sought. It may refuse. So be it.

WE ARE PART OF A LIVING PLANET

That notion of refusal is important. Plants and animals are not there for us. We exist as part of the web of life on a planet that is itself living. Other traditions have similar concepts. Ireland retains more than a flicker of its Celtic heritage. There, it's the faery folk and not devas who exist alongside plants – and woe betide you if you get on the wrong side of them. When American car manufacturer DeLorean came to Belfast, locals with an understanding of these things told the company not to take down a hawthorn tree on the site of the factory it was building. Greed trumped tradition, and the hawthorn was bulldozed. Within a year of the first car rolling off the line, the company was bankrupt.

Another aspect of this is the attitude of Britain to India in colonial days, something else Ireland has suffered from. The Irish had their language literally beaten out of them by the English. In India, many fragile palm leaf texts were taken home by members of the colonising forces, who saw quaint souvenirs in artefacts of a living tradition. Again, the belief that physical is all, and can exist out of context, in a display cabinet at home or the British Museum.

It's easy to extrapolate from that colonial tradition to how Ayurveda is often presented in the commercial arena, promoted as yet another panacea by frequently interchangeable influencers, though often their good intent is not matched by skills and depth of understanding. Intent is vital, and I use that term in its sense of connected to life force. The same can't always be said of what frequently happens within the pharmaceutical and health and beauty worlds, which tend to be more about profit and ownership above all else. Having been in meetings with them, this is something I've seen at first hand. For them, Ayurveda is another flavour of the week to be milked while the fad lasts. There'll be another one along soon enough – though whether the culture it's taken from will still exist in anything like a viable form is another question.

MISMATCH

Somewhere along the way, our relationship with planet has been skewed. Place and community used to come first, with the ways that we ebb and flow with them impossible to categorise and pin down because every instant is both a thing in its own right, and part of a web that's woven through time and space and genetics and culture.

In those universal traditions, the living world was recognised for what it was, with variations from place to place. Rivers were seen as entities in their own right. One win in recent years has been that in parts or all of some countries – India, New Zealand, Canada – rivers are once again acknowledged in that way. It's a triumph of campaigning by indigenous communities and activist allies, one that presents a welcome obstacle to a very different worldview.

That change matters because the ability of corporations to pollute and abuse waters that belong to none of us has led to environmental crimes on a global scale. For a river to be healthy, it needs to be able to cope with what flows through its waters. In Britain, dung containing high levels of nutrients from food for cows, pigs, and chickens is flushed into rivers by farmers because of a simple sum that they do. It's too expensive to transport the waste somewhere it can be disposed of, because the waste has no value. Viewed in financial terms, that's kind of true. But the consequences for waterways are drastic.

Plants which provide opportunities for young fish to grow in safety have been depleted in the River Wye by as much as 90%-97%. Any surviving plants are suffocated by algae blooming and related fungi. That in turn means no photosynthesis is happening. And without the cycle of carbon dioxide turning to oxygen, and vice versa it's not just the waters that suffer. What will we breathe? You can see more about the River Wye story in the documentary *Rivercide*. https://www.youtube.com/watch?v=5ID0VAUNANA Similar stories can be told worldwide.

Any of this is only possible in a world where those who hold power worship money and what they believe it can do for them above all else. A corporation exists to create shareholder value. That was the testament of economist Milton Friedman, whose views held sway over many governments for decades, starting with the Reagan era. As has been noted, were that corporation to be an individual, they would be a sociopath. Never mind cutesy logos and ads with ukulele soundtracks, think Hannibal Lecter.

IT'S YOUR TURN

This is about history. Family history. Yours.

Maybe you have answers for most or some of the questions that come up. If not, think who you could ask that might be able to share photos, anecdotes, and more.

1. In childhood, how much time did you spend outside? What kind of outside was that? Did it mean a local park at the weekend? A playing field at school? Relatives in the country or abroad you could visit from time to time?
2. Was 'outside' somewhere you felt happy and comfortable? Was it a special treat? Was it a regular and frequent part of your experience?
3. How old were you when you got a sense of where food came from?
4. When did you realise there was a connection between plants and herbs you were aware of, and meals and medicine?
5. Who was the first person you knew who grew vegetables or fruit or herbs? Was this a normal part of how and where you grew up, or something only a small number of people did?
6. Do you know the names of many plants? Do you wish you knew more about them, as well as their names? How many people your age have that kind of knowledge versus your impressions of who knew those things when you were a child?

SOIL BETWEEN YOUR TOES

You've probably heard of forest bathing. It's cropped up in articles and videos for a while now. The newest oldest thing. As a species, forests are part of our evolutionary journey. Folk stories the world over feature people going into or coming out of woods and encountering those – human, animal, and neither (elves and gnomes, leprechauns and brownies, etc) - that live there.

Being able to grow your own food, fruit, herbs, vegetables is one way to connect with ancestors. Your own, who tilled soil or foraged. And those in the area you live who did likewise at some point in the past, whatever your neighbourhood looks like now. And you can do it on a surprisingly small scale. A plantpot on the window of a seventh floor flat can grow something new, however much concrete and steel and glass are around.

The joy and frustration of being a grower is never quite knowing what's going to happen. Maybe your soil isn't ideal for what you had in mind, and you'll need to learn about composting. Some random insects might get to your harvest before you do. The seeds you were given might not actually be the ones you thought they were, and you end up with a mystery crop.

Whatever else your gardening adventure includes, I want to encourage you to cultivate a medicinal herb garden that will support you to create Ayurvedic results in a British climate. This chapter will not and is not intended to make you a herbalist. It is very much intended as a basic introduction, to spark inspiration for those who want to take this rewarding path further. If you are interested in making steps in that direction as part of your broader interest in Ayurveda and health, to the point where taking formal training will be advantageous, the material presented in the pages that follow will be useful.

START SIMPLE

We'll look at growing your own plants and making medicines from them more soon. It's always good to work with what's at hand, and at this point ginger is something that's easy to access in Britain. And its properties around health have long been known.

Jenya Di Pierro shares my passion for educating people about health and wellbeing and is one of the founders of the Cloud Twelve Lifestyle Club and Spa in Notting Hill. She kindly offered some of her recipes for ways that you can easily (and tastily) incorporate gnarly chunks of ginger into your and your family's medicine chest.

Ginger tea

Shredded ginger (it's up to you whether you remove the outer skin) steeped in boiling water for 3-5 minutes, with honey stirred in, is good for reliving throat soreness – and kills germs. Helpful for stomach ulcers and menstrual cramps too. It activates T-cells in your blood, which are active in dispelling viruses and protect you from disease.

Ginger candy

Boosts cognitive performance and memory – great before exams or presentations. And in candied form ginger is a yummy treat you can carry around and share with friends. You can achieve similar if less tasty effect by using ginger essential oil in a diffuser and letting the aroma do its work.

Candida cleanse with ginger

The causes of having an excess of candida (a yeast parasite we need some of...but only so much) include unhealthy diet. Symptoms include bloating, fatigue, acid reflux, and sugar craving. Juice an inch of ginger root and half a lemon, adding to water to drink as a tonic.

Golden latte

Not a ginger drink as such, but the ingredient that gives this drink its colour – turmeric – is a relative, and there's some ginger in here too. You'll want half a teaspoon of turmeric per cup, and just a touch each of ground ginger, ground cinnamon, and cayenne pepper. Add to your choice of warmed milk, and if you want to sweeten it add honey or stevia.

PLANTS AND PRINCIPLES

Ayurveda is about principles more than specifics where medicine is concerned: always choose a local plant that has a similar effect if an Indian one won't grow here. The aim is always results, not purism. And in some ways such an outcome is more straightforward than it may sound, given that herbs can be usefully categorised according to their particular kind of health-increasing or disease reducing effect:

- Antimicrobial
- Antiviral
- Digestion-enhancing
- Immune-boosting
- Nourishing
- Respiratory

A partial list of herbs that grow in the UK of interest to prompt further research includes:

- Aloe vera – good for dealing with constipation, and digestion generally.

- Burdock – a blood cleaner that stimulates digestion.
- Dandelion – useful for liver problems, jaundice, hepatitis, and ulcers.
- Echinacea – another blood cleanser, and good for lymph issues.
- Fennel seeds - great with indigestion, abdominal pain, difficulty or pain urinating.
- Garlic -for colds and coughs, skin disease, cholesterol and hypertension.
- Hawthorn berries – useful for circulatory and digestive problems.
- Juniper berries – active against arthritis, rheumatism, lumbago and sciatica.
- Liquorice root – useful for sore throats, heartburn, abdominal pain.
- Marshmallow – potent for coughs, bronchitis, kidney and bladder inflammation.
- Mint – soothes sore throats, reduces fever, headaches, and nervous upsets.
- Parsley – long used with gall stones, kidney stones, swollen breasts.
- Pennyroyal – valuable for menstrual cramps, headaches, and fevers.
- Raspberry leaves – used for uterine bleeding, inflamed mucus membranes, sores.

Some herbs have particular effects on individual organs, e.g. bladder, liver, or lungs. So where will you find the plants you need? A reputable nursery is your ally here. Let them know your interest is in medicinal grade herbs, rather than those which are either standard garden or ornamental varieties. A good nursery will be able to answer questions regarding to soil conditions, exposure, and climate as they affect outdoor plants. Some can be grown indoors of course, which may prompt questions from the nursery about which direction your window faces.

Alternatively, you could choose to forage wild herbs. The critical rule here is 100% certainty that you're picking what you hope to pick. If you're not quite sure the leaf shapes are as depicted in photographs, that it seems rather bigger than a guide indicates, leave it where it is. Time spent with a herbalist or forager who understands medicinal herbs can be a wise investment.

Make sure too that the plant is healthy. If you're interested in it supporting your vitality, why would you want a scrawny insect-riddled plant, unless you're confident of your abilities to revive it in your own garden?

RULES OF THUMB FOR THE HERB-GATHERER

- Use air-tight containers – boxes or zippable plastic bags.
- Label and date what you find using a pen that won't run.
- Only store leaves which have no discolouration (it's not about the look – it can indicate disease).

Already then, you can get a sense of the matrix of possibilities. You're suffering from a minor digestive upset, and there are three herbs at your disposal that could impact that. One of them also has an effect on the bladder, which given a secondary urinary aspect to what you're experiencing makes it a doubly effective route to pursue with some further consideration. The next question is one of formulation: how you will ingest or apply the herb, which is also a question of preparation.

Formulation:

- Tincture – in alcohol, vinegar, or glycerine.
- In creams and ointments for use on the skin.
- Infused oils.
- Syrups.
- Tonic wines.
- Dried – for use as a herbal tea or infusion.
- Powder – loose or in capsules.
- Poultices and compresses.

KITCHEN SINK PHARMA

You'll need to be suitably stocked up with a variety of equipment to head in a herbalist direction. Bear that in mind ahead of time. What you already have might do the job, but better now you have an appropriate kit than be forced to improvise with unknown consequences.

Kitchen/cookware
- Pots, pans.
- Drying racks.

- Tea kettle.
- Teapot (ceramic for natural heat retention).
- Glass or ceramic bowls.
- Tea strainers in different sizes.
- Funnels.
- Measuring cups, measuring and regular spoons, spatulas, whisks...

Storage and usage

- Jars or tins with tight-fitting lids.
- Different size glass jars suitable for preserving food.
- Different size and colour bottles with lids, including ones with droppers.
- Labels.
- Cotton balls or cosmetic pads.

CAUTIONS

Prepared properly by someone who knows what they're doing, herbal remedies can be life-changing. The key words there are "someone who knows what they're doing". Consider how many people do a course, are enthusiastic for a few months or make it a background part of the person they think they want to be for years, compared with the number who really put the work in to make that dream come true. Now ask yourself which of them you'd trust when offered a soothing herbal tonic which will set you right. And be real about your own progress if you do set that goal for yourself. Lives are at stake.

The importance of labelling has already been mentioned. Backing labels up with a written and photographic record can be helpful to be able to identify just what was picked, what it looked like at the time, and what was done with it. Given the potential consequences of a herbal remedy interacting with a prescribed pharmaceutical someone didn't tell you they were taking, or provoking an allergic reaction, being meticulous assumes new levels of significance.

IT'S YOUR TURN

This chapter has been written intentionally to make the path of growing medicinal herbs and utilising them correctly a little daunting. And it's also the case that you've taken on many challenges in your life successfully that require research and planning and the development of new skills. Some questions to point you to those resources and how you can use them in this context:

1. What's a good example of something you've done that involved learning new practical skills?
2. How did you approach that task, and what about it will be useful in nurturing your skills with herbs and preparing them into preparations with health benefits?
3. What are your research skills like? How many sources do you consult when you're learning about something new?
4. Who do you know who could introduce you to some of the skills and knowledge you're hoping to acquire?
5. Do you know a reputable nursery in your area? Who would be a good person to ask if not?
6. Given the amount of room you have to grow herbs, and the need to bring new equipment into your kitchen, drawing up a plan that starts small and grows to a manageable size would be good.
7. If you were to team up with some friends or relatives for this adventure, who would be good to ensure a balanced set of outlooks and experience?
8. What could you do right now to make the first step in this new direction?

THINKING THINGS AND EXTENDED THINGS

MEDITATION | YOGA | TANTRA

We know that cultures worldwide found ways to feed themselves and in addition use some of the foods they enjoyed in supporting their recovery from a wide range of ailments and injuries. That's the case whether you're in Africa, Latin America, Europe, Japan...it's a prerequisite for a civilisation that it develops means of keeping people healthy.

The particulars of how that works will vary from one region to another. It's inevitable, for the simple reason that plant populations shift according to soil type, climate, altitude, and more. The word used by the French for this is *terroir* – it's for this reason that wine is so important to the French. What one vineyard grows can be different in nuanced ways from another just a few miles away.

For the Italians too, it's a similar story. Regional dishes vary not just from one village to another, but within families, and there is justified pride in that distinctiveness. When you're welcomed to a home to share a meal, listening to the story of how the pork tastes like that because of acorns the wild pigs eat in a near-by forest, you're dining not just with those around the table, but their ancestors.

Something happened to change that recognition of the importance of land and community, and its roots are there in Descartes and his elevation of mind over nature. As organisms using verbal language, he supposed we were smarter than other creatures we share the planet with. Having a cat in the house would have made him question that assumption: Descartes believed animals operate purely by reflex. And many of those who followed in that line were fond not just of the human faculty for thought, but the specific ideas of people like themselves, who could intellectualise in similar fashion. A pity – two centuries before him, fellow Frenchman Montaigne recognised cats can play, and are self-aware rather than purely responsive to what happens around them.

A key distinction Descartes made was the concept of *thinking things*. This referred to people – not all of them, though. He didn't credit animals with awareness or ascribe it to all humans either. All the better to exploit them – which is where *extended things* comes in. Extended things are seen in his fundamentally broken outlook as being subject to the whim of thinkers. For instance, indigenous peoples required to extract minerals from their own land to create profit for those brighter than them.

Francis Bacon, 16th century English scientist and also the country's Attorney General and Lord Chancellor, paved the way for Descartes in some respects, expressed this perspective with brutal clarity: "science should as it were torture nature's secrets out of her." Read that quote again. Notice the 'her' and ponder its connection with 200,000 women killed in Europe between the 1480s and 1750 because they were supposedly witches. What that meant in practice was women who knew about herbal lore, midwifery, and other lore that women shared between them.

These are the attitudes that paved the way for the reordering of humankind's relationship with the planet we live on. It's done for the benefit of that minuscule numbers of those – mostly men - who can turn natural resources into a pleasing number of zeroes on their bank accounts so that they can sleep at night. As for the rest of us...well, never mind. We're just more extended things.

WETIKO, HUNGRY GHOSTS, AND ILLTH

If we're going to come up with unusual wordings like 'extended things', let's see where we can find some more helpful ones. One is *wetiko*. This is a concept of the Cree tribe of Native Americans. Wetiko describes how people conduct themselves that takes them from beyond the normal social orbit and defines them as predators. Wetiko is about taking from others and hoarding what's taken though the thief could never possibly make use of what they've stolen. It's a disorder the Cree see in spiritual terms and can be thought of as a virus that we all have to some degree.

It's not fanciful to argue the Cree had a healthier outlook in part because their society was focused on individual and collective wellbeing. They had a notion of what a socially healthy individual was like, and a structure of initiations involving community support for their people as they progressed from one stage of life to another. That concern was ongoing and inclusive. Western societies lack such a formal framework for guidance, and instead devote resources to the consequences of not having one. Prisons, mental hospitals, and facilities for substance abuse are a brutal and loveless substitute for failure to care for people properly in the first place. And they make a lot of money for those running them.

Another take on the phenomenon of compulsive acquisition with people seen purely in terms of their worth as economic assets comes from Buddhism. Stories are told about hungry ghosts. These are beings with endless appetite, but only a pinprick sized mouth to take in sustenance. As such, they're forever starved, while living in a world of plenty.

We live in a world of hungry ghosts. And we've all been among their number, longingly looking at videos of an even better car, a more desirable pair of shoes, the holiday of a lifetime.

A third term that may be new to you: *illth*. It's borrowed from Victorian thinker John Ruskin - art critic, philanthropist, and social thinker. Where wealth points to the benefits of accruing artefacts, property, land, and money, illth takes into the account the downside that necessarily accompanies such acquisition.

Illth can be seen in environmental damage and the effects on employees of working with toxic substances. It can be experienced socially too. Long-established British bed manufacturers Silentnight were sold to private equity group HIG in a way that meant taxpayers would pick up the bill for the company's 1200 pension-holders, who've not had access to the financial support they spent their working lives building up. This chicanery was organised by a senior member of leading accountancy firm KPMG, who also worked with HIG. The firm has been fined for its misdeeds, but some former workers will be dead before their pensions are recovered.

USE THE FORCE

Back in the nineteenth century, there was a point when hypnosis was used to prepare patients for surgery. One of the big names in the field was John Elliotson, who opened The London Mesmeric Infirmary in 1849 and performed operations including amputations. And there were others, people like James Esdaile, who did 300 major and 100 minor operations using hypnosis.

Around the same time, nitrous oxide was gaining popularity. A learned committee looked into hypnosis and declared it bogus, saying that patients were just pretending not to feel pain when they had their limbs hacked off. It later transpired that these statements were falsified, but by then it was too late for hypnosis in the mainstream. If you're in the business of supplying nitrous oxide – or other alternatives - you've got a profitable incentive to discredit the opposition.

Franz Anton Mesmer, who the London Mesmeric Infirmary was named after, was an 18th century doctor who believed in a phenomenon he called animal magnetism. His ideas about the subject lean in the direction of astrology and energy, the former a conversation-stopper for some, and the latter a nebulous word for good measure. Which isn't to say that it lacks value. The inability to specify precisely what form of energy is involved doesn't prevent a conversation where both parties can agree that a something happened to them or between them.

Next time someone raises an eyebrow about the subject, ask them to explain the nature of what happens when they make love. Is it best explained with diagrams and measuring aids, or the shared experience of being intimate, which varies every time and at its best has something miraculous beyond the scope of the laboratory? Definitely nothing to do with animal magnetism, or chi, or prana, or any of the other terms that peoples worldwide have used to articulate something about the essence of being human...

Mesmer is conveniently dead, and those who speak of him at all label his work under the heading of hypnosis, which is a more generally acceptable way to refer to influence and hence language. In doing so we're back in Descartes territory, since manipulating people through words on behalf of those seeking to exploit them was becoming a science of its own by the start of the twentieth century. Part of the reason was Freud. And staying with language and ideas is a convenient way of putting to one side the bigger issue of energy in wellbeing, which always seems connected with three human universals: breath, movement, and attention.

One figure who wasn't done with the notion of energy, someone hard to categorise from a conventional perspective, is Wilhelm Reich. A student of Freud's, Reich got interested in life force and sexuality and the ways it's shaped by the societies we live in. Wherever and whenever people have lived, there have been codes concerning what is or is not acceptable for two or more when they meet with sexual intent. Church or state are in the bedroom, and Reich wasn't convinced they had any business being there.

The researcher worked at the point Hitler was emerging from the catastrophe of post-WW1 Germany. Out of that experience came his book *The Mass Psychology of Fascism*. It didn't go down well (nor with the communists there) and the psychologist's work was burned in his home-country. Fleeing to America, the same happened. Six tons of Reich's books were burned, and he died there in prison in 1956.

MONOPOLY MEDICINE

It says much that two powerful nations were so vehemently opposed to Reich's concepts about how the state warps the development and expression of healthy individuals. A similar pattern can be seen in how the centuries-old practice of natural medicine in the west was eroded to allow powerful wealthy men to acquire greater power and wealth.

Those two men were America's original billionaire, oil tycoon John D. Rockefeller and his friend steel magnate Andrew Carnegie. Seeing the potential to involve oil and its by-products in the creation of medicines, in 1910 the prestigious Carnegie Foundation sent Andrew Flexner to do a report on the country's medical colleges and hospitals. He was unimpressed by what he found – and in some cases he was justified…America's 'snake oil' and 'quack doctor' tradition exists for good reasons. But principally the methods he came across were rooted in herbalism, bodywork, and more, with European and Native American influences – which people had returned to for generations. The Spanish flu epidemic of 1918 strengthened the zeal of Rockefeller's campaign against forms of medicine he wasn't going to see profit from.

As a result of Flexner's report, half of the country's 166 medical colleges that existed in 1904 gradually became 76 by 1930. Those that survived did so thanks to injections of cash in the form of grants to stop them teaching the now-discredited old model, removing any reference to herbs and nutrition, and offer instead the allopathic approach to medicine. All taught the same curriculum. This drove a greater move to surgery, along with bloodletting and the use of lead and mercury injections to flush out disease.

Along with this, an extensive media campaign demonised the older ways. Newspaper articles as well as advertising conveyed your parents and grandparents were wrongheaded with their quaint stories about the poultices and potions that kept them healthy or helped them recover when they weren't. Some doctors were even jailed for prescribing medicines used safely and effectively for decades.

Over time, Rockefeller saw the key to his strategy was removing nature from medicine. If people could grow herbs locally or access someone in their area who could help them get better, he was missing out on dollars. The artificial synthesis of vitamin C in Switzerland in 1935 presented the prospect of a future where medicines were produced in labs. As such they were patentable - meaning more money for Rockefeller and his allies. Buying a chunk of the German drug company I.G. Farben gave him a foothold into the market, and pretty soon the new 'pill for every ill' model was up and running.

After John D. Rockefeller's death successors in his business attempted in the 1960s to make it impossible for natural health approaches to be used in countries that were members of the United Nations. Instead, billions of people would be required to use the medications created by pharmaceutical companies following the allopathic model. Fortunately those attempts were thwarted to an extent, but the path since then has been one of extending a fundamentally toxic acquisitive influence worldwide.

Now, in 2021, the Rockefeller Foundation aims to achieve Health For All by working with partners internationally. Recently the Foundation pledged $13.5m to act against what they term "confusing, inaccurate and harmful" information about health. Some things never change.

AND THERE IS HOPE

Awareness of the facts about how modern medicine came to be is useful. And bear in mind too of the incredible benefits it's created for people across the globe. Polio has barely been a problem in much of the world for nearly a century. Longevity has increased worldwide. Couples with fertility problems are having babies that would have been impossible without IVF. Developments in cardiac surgery save countless people from heart issues that were typically a fast track to an early death. Contraception has given women more control of their lives in a way that's changed society and economy. And so forth. There are many reasons for gratitude, not to be forgotten.

Before all those welcome advances - and beyond the realm of allopathic medicine or herbal preparations - there were millennia where cultures worldwide had ways to work with breath, movement, and attention to ensure their wellbeing. Many were developed and refined in the living tradition of Ayurveda in the practices of yoga, meditation, and tantra.

Without breath, there is nothing. Look at the word *respiration*. Those four letters *spir* have their origins in *spirit*. And you'll see them too in inspiration. Go back to Middle English and its meaning was *"breathe or put life or spirit into the human body; impart reason to a human soul."* And in Ayurveda, the same recognition exists. It's what ties yoga, meditation, and tantra together. *Prana* means *life force*, and breath is the chief way in which we it and can work with it.

MEDITATING ON MEDITATION

How we breathe affects mind and body. Actually, let's use the term body-mind to get away from the wrongness of 'I think therefore I am'. We are whole beings. And at this point let's explore what that means for us.

At the moment you're reading this text. Which means some of your attention is here, on these words. *Hi, how are you doing?* Maybe that question made you smile, and maybe it leads you to notice something about the place you're reading or reflect on how your day has gone so far. And it's possible that the way you feel has shifted because of what happened when your attention went to those other facets of your reality.

Sometimes those shifts happen of their own accord through something unexpected. Two days ago, a friend came around to my house with an angle grinder to cut up scraps of metal making them easier to dispose. The angle grinder cast furious sparks around the space as he worked. And within 20 minutes he was gone, back into his van and away again.

The oddity of the experience struck me more as the day went. And reminded me that houses are often seen as representing the mind by psychologists and those interested in dreams. For a while, I'd welcomed an intrusive element into mine – who did something valuable and then went.

Last night, I went to visit a client I've become friendly with. In truth, after a demanding day I wasn't in a mood to 'perform' for new people, which was my expectation. Instead, the evening took a different turn. My client had to get involved with tense last-minute communications with the aggressive business man buying a company her father founded. I got to spend time with father and daughter, individually and together, over the course of the evening. In doing so, far from that sense of wearing a social mask we all sometimes experience, I got to listen and engage with them in ways I'd never have done had we sat eating food together as expected.

In the second scenario, I was witness to dramas occurring under someone else's roof, easier to be reflective about that than your own trials and tribulations. That enabled me to be of use for a family anxious about the effect of the business buyer's unjustifiably hostile behaviour on a dad looking forward to retirement.

All of this is in the realm of attention. And as with houses that may also be our mind, so too with the ways our bodies work. That tension in your ribs you notice some days more than others. The stab of pain that when you put a particular pair of shoes on which you tolerate. A high hum in your ears sometimes which may be tinnitus but can mostly be left alone, even appreciated for the way it permeates the sounds of nature.

SIMPLE STEPS ON A LIFELONG PATH

Meditation is the art, and science, and discipline, that allows us to work with attention. Over time it becomes something to peer both outside and in, and to get a sense of how the interior and external worlds reflect one another.

Think of the house stories as metaphors about how attention works, and the stories you get caught up in, and meditation as a way to give you more choices about your roles in them. Begin go recognise your patterns as they emerge and they will change. Become familiar with the workings of bodymind to spot that a stray thought is no more than words cut and pasted from past experience bearing no relation to now. Breathing life into your thoughts and feelings restores your connection with self and nature, and the reality that they – we - are one.

A good place to start with meditation, and one you can always return to, is with doing something simple and repetitive to keep yourself partly occupied and free some of your attention up for self-awareness. It's why *mantras* are used: simple repetitive phrases. *Mandalas* – images that are geometrically constructed – have a similar effect, giving the eyes something to look at. And focusing on breath also has function, though there's a lot more to breathing than a rhythm to focus on. Of course, the same can be said for mantras and mandalas.

Choosing to meditate with intent will give you greater insight into the ways bodymind functions:

The itch that starts on your arm 20 minutes into a 30 minute sitting meditation.

The pride you have in achieving an hour of meditation which gets you onto a spiral about how pride is bad and you need to start again.

The resentment you feel for both the comment and the suggestion.

The amusement when you realise all those reactions happened in you.

Much of international meditation teacher Davidji's work is rooted in experience of the here and now. This Drishti Meditation comes from his book *Secrets of Meditation*, one of my favourites. Throughout, use a fixed gaze with soft eyes.

Take a deep breath, hold it in for a few beats. And then slowly let it out through your nostrils. Keep breathing at this same pace. Long, slow, deep inhales.

After you've done this a few times, drift your gaze to the tip of your nose. Feel your eyes cross and relax. Do this for a minute or so.

Now bring your awareness up to your third eye, located in the middle of your forehead, a bit above your eyebrows. Feel your eyes open and close. Stay in this space for a few minutes.

Now bring your attention to your navel. Look within. Keep your eyes in a soft gaze. Stay here for a few minutes.

And now gently drift your thumbs-no thoughts but your gaze for a few minutes.

And now expand your awareness to include your whole hand. Keep breathing ... long ... slow ... deep breaths.

Now drift your gaze to your big toes. Wiggle them to bridge the energetic distance between your physical and astral toes.

Now without moving your head, drift your gaze all the way to the right, almost trying to see your right ear. Keep your gaze soft, and keep breathing.

Now move your ears as far as they will gaze in the other direction.

After you've gazed left for a minute or so, bring the gaze to the centre and raise your eyes up to the sky.

When you've done that for a minute or so, close your eyes and just sit and let that process settle in.

After you've practiced that meditation, or before it depending on your inclination and schedule, check out the following sequence that may help illuminate what you experienced during the Davidji process. These are useful pointers for many situations, especially if you're feeling stressed or anxious...

IT'S YOUR TURN

Sitting down, spend a minute to check in with your thoughts. Just let them pass.

How much of your mind is words, and how much images and sounds and feelings?

How about your body? Starting with your neck and shoulders, where do you notice tension?

Scanning through your chest and abdomen, how are they?

What about your back and limbs?

How is your breathing right now?

If you can let yourself suspend judgement, then do so. Much of what passes through us is judgement in one form or another. We're human. It's fine. Don't judge yourself for it.

YOGΛ – IT'S MORE THΛN YOU THINK

Meditation is part of yoga, and yoga can be a tool for meditation. The boundaries matter less than the experience. It's akin to being asked about a bottle that you're looking at: is it green, or is it glass? Well, it's both.

You'll have some sense of yoga already. And may well practice it regularly or at least have some experience. The fact it's so pervasive, bringing up thoughts about everything from yoga mats to controversial schools of yoga, gets in the way of what yoga was intended to be. The name yoga itself means union, its aim to cultivate good health through practices encouraging physical health and flexibility, emotional stability and good mental hygiene. All of that in turn strengthens the immune system, which will be good for whatever adventures are ahead of you.

Any yoga routines and workouts you'll be aware of to whatever extent are a means of finding that kind of equilibrium. Our physical, mental, and emotional aspects are different colours of the same bottle. And western science increasingly backs up the contention that bodymind is one. Genetics established the connection between physical and other traits that we inherit from our parents and pass onto our children. And we now have increasing evidence for the impact that trauma can have on our descendants, thanks to the science of epigenetics.

For many people the emphasis on physical yoga as a means of keeping in trim, with a side order of mindfulness, is just what they're looking for. As such, it's to be appreciated. Anything that helps people get by in a world as chaotic as ours is very welcome.

And there's more. From an Ayurvedic perspective, yoga offers tools for the development of spirit. Or put another way, and again make use of that valuable western perspective, one description of what yoga offers is the prospect of liberation from at least some consequences of our genetic and epigenetic inheritance, for ourselves and what we transmit to future generations. But doing that requires more than what's presented as yoga in nearly all cases. We need to look further. We need to experience *tantra*.

TANTRA, AND MONKEY BUSINESS

There comes a point, when you've lived with Ayurveda for a while, when meditation and yoga are part of your daily existence, that a shift happens. You may notice it as a feeling of liberation when you appreciate your often robotic responses to the world are part of a web woven through your life. Every moment can present the realisation you are both the spider and the fly on that web, the web itself, and are none of them and all of them simultaneously. Or you may wake up one morning, and for no readily apparent reason have an awareness of yourself as a shard of something divine.

For me, part of that journey was an unexpected glimpse of a bigger context on a ten-day silent retreat. I'd gone knowing I was in need to time out, to let my body show me who I was again, to be free of what was happening with and to and around and for me at that point. Every day we would rise to be ready for a 5.30 meditation, and that plus meals was pretty much the routine.

Seven days in, I found myself crying.

There's an expression of Freud's. "We leak the truth through every pore." I was leaking then for sure. I didn't know what truth was coming out, but my body was letting go of something. Now when I think of that quote, what comes to mind is "We pour the truth through every leak."

I cried. And I found myself. Not all of me. And not all at once. But something shifted.

That was an experience of tantra in action, a way to consider and experience the awakening of the soul and become aware of the blockages we have at an energetic level. With that ability we have the capacity to experience freedom which is the root of spontaneity, confidence, and connection. And living with them more often, we discover faith based not on any text but on the recognition we are now living differently.

To comprehend tantra, consider everything you experience as food. The tv shows you watch, the gossip you listen to, the clothes you choose, the decisions you opt for and the ones you turn from. All of them go into creating the potential for a cosmic entity in the 80,000 or so days we're likely to be on this planet. They're transformed into nutrients to sustain us on our way. And every now and then we need to dispose of some of it. At which point, like me, you too might burst in tears 70% of the way through a process that was ~~way~~ acting like a pressure cooker for everything I was holding.

If you want to see someone who is alive with energy in the ways tantra opens, think of the comedian and actor Robin Williams. There was a magic about him which was beautifully simple. He was open to the moment, and to the people and context he was in wherever he happened to be. You can see it in his performances, his improvisations, and the way he engaged with Koko, a gorilla taught sign language to communicate with humans. After the death of her mate, Robin Williams was the first person to make Koko happy again. And when the comedian died, the gorilla mourned him.

Tantra is about the awakening of the soul, and the realisation that we are cosmic beings. Our sense of what cosmic might entail will change over time, because why wouldn't it? And part of that path is about finding balance within the female and male aspects of yourself, and with those you come across. Opening the door to tantra changes everything.

IT'S YOUR TURN

What's it like, in your head most of the time?

No. Really. What's it like being in your head?

How much of what you do on a day-by-day basis supports your wellbeing?

How much of your thought and behaviour is you, and how much is a result of the roles you've chosen or been conditioned to play?

Have you had a glimpse of another life that matters enough to you to pursue it?

Yes? How's it going? Be honest.

In the final section of the book you'll find a piece enabling you to work out what your dosha is. With that knowledge you will also be able to check out the yoga postures illustrated and work with those which are a good match.

IT'S IN THE MEΛT

HANDS-ON THERAPY

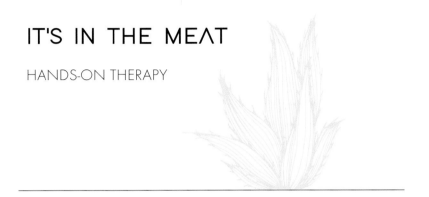

I'm going to shock you in a small and well-intentioned way. And there's a good reason for that. Ayurveda has existed for millennia, and the world it exists in has changed beyond measure. To some extent, Ayurveda too has changed – at the very least in its presentation. The sages who wrote some of the earliest material we know didn't have Instagram accounts, for one thing, or feel pressured to do sexy yoga poses for their followers. Part of my intent with this book is to bridge that gap between the ancient, the contemporary, and what's yet to come. So with that in mind, here's a core something it's good to be reminded of:

We are animals.

Many writers and practitioners of disciplines we call spiritual are inclined to make the same mistake as Descartes did around mind and assume spirit and body are separate. They're not. We are spirits in suits of flesh that are easily bruised or punctured, hung on bones which can break, kept going by organs needing sustenance, and with awareness of the world constructed through overlapping maps derived from our senses. Get up at night to use the toilet and bump a knee on a door that your eye hasn't registered fully. Next morning the same route will be clear, even if you've no memory about why your knee is now sore.

You can't separate spirit from body any more than you could remove the colour from your favourite shoes. They are one. Even if you practice or believe in astral projection or remote viewing, even if you've had a near-death experience, all of that only counts if you've got a living body waiting to return to after that jaunt.

Our meat matters. Everything we do and everything we can be is that way because we are embodied. It couldn't be otherwise. Never mind being ignorant of other dimensions - if you're not tall enough you won't even know what's on top of a wardrobe. Without going to Wales, no amount of tv shows about the country will convey that experience. It might as well be Narnia. And if that's true of Wales, what are we to make of news about Afghanistan? It's being somewhere, which also necessarily means being rooted in time, that allows us to experience the universe in our unique way.

Whatever we don't experience directly is speculation, and so too is much of what we make of our own lives. How often have you mistaken a stranger for a friend? I don't mean that in any wafty cosmic way. No, I mean looking across the road and seeing your friend Casey – that's her for sure, going on colour and style hair, height, and dress sense. Only, she seems to be avoiding your call and wave. Hmm, rude. So you cross over the road to let her know what a fake she is only for Casey to open her mouth and...words come out with the wrong accent. From a face without Casey's freckles. And a body shorter than you where Casey is taller. Welcome to Beth.

Finding your centre...or centres...

In that incident – and we've all experienced variations – there's a mix of things going on. The tradition represented by Armenian mystic Gurdjieff has a handy way of accounting for them, and methods for dealing with such tangled experiences of the everyday more effectively through thinking of ourselves anew. There are parallels in other systems, Ayurveda included.

Viewed through the lens Gurdjieff used, people have three centres: a movement centre, a thinking centre, and a feeling centre. We need all of them, and each has its own capabilities, preferred form of nourishment, and potential for going out of kilter.

- In that instance then, you saw a woman across the road, and gambled on a first glance that this was a friend. *Thinking centre: all sensory impressions are gambles until validated.*

- Tried and failed to attract her attention. *Movement and emotion centres.*
- Annoyed by imaginary rudeness, you walked through traffic to give her a piece of the mind you weren't using, discovering you'd make the journey as the result of an error. *All three centres, actively engaged in a mission that could have resulted in a hospital trip.*

It's a hop and a skip away from three centres to seven chakras, among other maps useful for comprehending and working with human capability. And bodywork is a great way not just to restore lost capacity - in the case of remedial massage - but to unlock the possibilities that exist at the other side of trauma. Sometimes trauma is very evident, in the aftermath of a loved one's death, or the experience of a serious accident or injury. It can also reside in forms that we often believe don't merit the term trauma and hence are less inclined to do something about. Childhood dreams dismissed by a busy teacher's offhand remark, a colleague's strategically hurtful comment, the suffering of a beloved pet.

A great way to get to know the world better is by being kind to ourselves, a big part of which is understanding and maintaining our animal - all the better to relish life for many years to come. Reach back into your memory and you will discover the taste of soil, what your gran's table looked like from underneath, how gravel feels on your knees when you fall off a bike. Since your earliest days you've been learning about the world and what you know is encoded in every fibre and facet of you. And some of the knowledge you carry with is faulty.

I remember the first time we went to the seaside as a family. We sat on a blanket, and I enjoyed an ice cream. The sea was there, and I perhaps understood it was bigger than anything I'd seen before. Maybe almost as big as the sky it was beneath. At some point I got up and took a step off the blanket. And shrieked. The ground shifted. Nobody told me this was a thing that happened. It probably hadn't occurred to my parents it was something I'd need to know. Or I didn't listen. Ground was firm. Ground being sand you could make impressions in and wiggle your toes between was alien.

IT'S YOUR TURN

Stand or sit comfortably and breathe in a way that makes you feel good. What experiences in your life have imprinted you with beliefs and feelings that limit you? Pick a minor example, something that's no more than 3 on a scale of 1-10.

When you bring that example to mind, what happens to your breathing? And to your thoughts and feelings?

Take a step or two away and breathe in a way that relaxes you.

Now, consider a good memory, one that helped give you something positive in life.

Enjoy those sensations, and after you've done so for a while notice what's different about your breathing and the way your body feels. How are your thoughts and emotions at this point?

ENERGY FLOWS WHERE ATTENTION GOES

Doing that exercise will have reminded you of something you're already very aware of. That how we feel and what we are capable of moment by moment is an endlessly changing stream of sensations. A lot of the time it's one that's fine to experience as it turns up. But there are points when you can spot that you're in or heading for a meltdown on some scale. And being able to work with your body in small or larger ways, alone or with assistance, provides great ways to steer yourself away from approaching rocks. Plus, who wouldn't want to feel fitter, healthier, and happier on an ongoing basis?

The cocktail of what's happened to you, the responses you have about it, and the conclusions you come to as a result, shape a lot of the person you become. And you will change even more over time because all of us age, some of us give birth, and we are all at risk of breaking limbs, losing more of our sensory capabilities than we may have imagined. All of which provide reasons to make sure we get to know and look after our bodies.

You may well have already found that yoga and massage can provide release at a deeper level than you anticipated and want to know more about how an Ayurvedic approach to those practices can support you further. And it can. Working with your body using the tools and knowledge Ayurveda provides allows partial or sometimes greater liberation from pain and at least some limitations, making possible a brighter future than you may have dreamed of before.

NOTHING IS ALL OR NOTHING

Dualities exist in the mind, and only then until they're challenged. An interest in Ayurveda and training in the lore and skills involved, does not preclude you from receiving conventional medical support where contextually it provides a better option. As someone with that expertise who has trained over a thousand people in them to a high standard, I'm grateful for the opportunities conventional medicine provides for the application of what we know in the service of patient wellbeing.

Surgical patients understandably experience sometimes considerable anxiety around the whole process of getting ready for an operation. Sometimes it requires weight loss, or specific changes in blood pressure or blood sugar to be attained before surgery is possible. The pressures involved can cause hypertension and affect pain thresholds and recovery time. Added to that, the logistical and bureaucratic aspects of it all are not for the fainthearted. For good measure, medications at any stage of all this may create unwanted effects, some of which may delay the operation and in turn add to the stresses the not-yet-patient goes through even before they reach the theatre.

No surprise then, that an article in *Complementary Therapies in Clinical Practice* (Volume 41, November 2020) drawing on 25 studies with almost 2500 patients, showed that massage reduces anxiety for most surgical patients. Massage using acupoints or targeting body reflex areas was more impactful for the resolution of anxiety than general massage. And in clinical settings, those massages worked best at 10-20 minutes.

The skilled application of fingers and oil we tend to think of it being relaxing and a release. Physiologically, what's happening is what we sense as tension going is about lactic acid and other waste products from muscles being expelled. Circulation is stimulated, blood pressure lowered, and digestion improved – not least because you'll be more inclined to excrete what's surplus. As well, endorphins released by touch will make you feel good and relax.

The effects of massage go beyond a lift in mood, welcome though that can be. A study in the *Journal of Cancer Survivorship* (December 2020) showed that patients – who often experience poor sleep because of the drugs they're prescribed – sleep for longer and feel better when they do thanks to massage.

That kind of objective data about sleep duration is valuable, but with such a personal and intimate experience you've really got to rely on your own response. If you feel better, you feel better. If that's not happening through someone's massage, they're probably not the person who should be doing it for you: the feedback is right at their fingertips, not in your words. And what they sense through those fingertips will vary according to what training and experience they are drawing on.

WHY AYURVEDIC MASSAGE IS DIFFERENT

Where Ayurveda is distinct from other forms of massage is in part around the extent to which it uses oils, and how and why they're used. And in turn that relates to the foundational concept of doshas, which is simultaneously the aspect of Ayurveda people feel they can explain in a soundbite, and the heart of a living and sophisticated multifaceted, complex, living body of knowledge stretching back thousands of years.

Doshas are an expression of the language of this ancient outlook that guides practitioners, but not the language itself. They are a way to understand how someone's physiology and emotions are different aspects of an individual, who is subject to the influence of food and weather and the impact of others. And to get a sense of what makes those distinctions and changes possible, we need to understand the underlying essence which allows doshas to be expressed.

A half-decent analogy might be that you're aware that different languages exist, that languages differ, and can express similar concepts and things in the world.

English: eggs

Hindi: अंडे

Mandarin: 蛋

Language itself, which can exist in many forms depending where and when you're hatched, is another matter. Developing an awareness of its essence takes time, experiencing people who speak different ones, and finding out how they communicate in the absence of shared written or spoken words. It's at that point you're getting to the essence which allows such a wide range of specific manifestations to exist. And in the context of Ayurveda and massage (and more) that essence is *prana*.

Prana is subtle, implicit in so much of what we already have names for, there without us even knowing. It's present in the doshas and the muscles and in yoga and in meditation and in herbs and food and more. And that presence is experienced throughout our bodies at subtle points akin to acupuncture points. They're known as *marmas*, and it's only because of prana's ever-shifting fluidity and ability to present in places we never expected, that we can get away with calling this next section of the chapter:

MARMA CHAMELEON

If you're going to be massaging someone, you'll be affecting their marma points. Given that, it will really help if you develop an understanding of them to finesse your Ayurvedic skills. With the ability to work with them and with knowledge of *nadis*, the channels through which prana travels, a skilled practitioner effectively has a London Underground map – nadis are the lines, and marmas are stations.

Prana is life force, is soul, the breath of creation as it unfolds in every instant. We can cultivate prana with the way we treat our bodies, and in what we eat and drink and through many other choices we make. We are never not relating to, processing, transmitting or receiving prana in some way or some form because prana is of the cosmos itself. It's the connective tissue (only not tissue) of how and why each and every individual reflects reality in their unique ways, every person's microcosm itself a macrocosm from head to feet, skin and bones, teeth and nails. Which if you're the sort of person who's unnecessarily humble provides a great reason to keep yourself in good shape: you're looking after the universe!

SKIN IS THE WAY IN

We're contained in a self-repairing multi-layered cellular envelope that does so much for us. It keeps our insides where they should be, guides our awareness of temperature and other environmental shifts, and is sensitive in different ways in different places. Try it. Find out what's the closest distance you can distinguish two points on your hand, and then discover what the equivalent space is beneath a knee. Our fingers and hands are used in so many ways and can pick up a rich array of sensory information. That gap between the knee and the foot? Not so much for most of us unless we've trained as a climber or dancer and pick up distinctions thanks to skin as well as the muscle that would not be apparent to most.

Be good to your skin, and it will be good to you. In Ayurveda terms, that means using oils that will complement your dosha. That's one of the areas in which Tri-Dosha has made impact. After I started to work with spas in 2008, I recognised the need for dosha-specific oils suited to the expectations of those working in spaces and their clients. Understanding Ayurveda, I could see how that would work – making a dozen and frequently more herbs grown on land where my grandfather first planted them and integrating them with herbs and oils native to Britain and Europe. Always the same principles, adapting to the culture of the day. Without it, the result is stagnation – no need to revive a tradition when it can be kept healthy.

Skin is the envelope in which we deliver ourselves to the world. Every day we are exposed to different surfaces and substances, some of them safe and others potentially hazardous. A beauty-focused approach to the use of massage and oils in skincare only goes so far...it's literally skindeep, and that's just the start of what's attainable. Think Grand Canyon. Tourists pose for a photo in front of the stunning view. The explorer gets down, maybe as far as the Colorado River, a walk of a few hours that many describe as a transformative experience. Ayurvedic massage provides that deep tissue alchemy – and will improve your complexion too.

The core of such massage is muscle. If you think of the term *muscle learning* you'll get why. We have an incredible array of habits and skills pretty much running by reflex. Along the way we may well have acquired bad habits.

And that applies to some of the very best in their field.

Tiger Woods redefined golfing brilliance twice. First in his unprecedented career up until 2005. And then with a comeback in 2019 when after a combination of physical injury and personal turmoil his life and career looked in jeopardy. To do that Woods needed to reinvent his approach to the inner and outer aspects of play, sculpting his body to explore and master a new way of doing what had already made him a world-beater.

SELF-MASSAGE

If you enjoy walking barefoot (and I hope you do) you'll be aware of the capacity it has to liven you up on even the dullest day. That may or may not be something to do with earth energies if you're inclined to such concepts, but for sure it's about having your soles massaged by the slow-to-yield solidity of uneven mud and stone and grass. Maybe that's where those earth energies get in, through the marmas. They'll give your tootsies a workout you'll benefit from for hours. Same goes for the delights of leaning against of a well-chosen tree and its day-changing effect on your spine and shoulders.

Even better, you can use oil and indulge yourself in an experience closer to the spa. A sesame oil base with herbs you know are right for you is a good place to start, and there are variations on this theme. Before you heat the oil (just above body temperature), get in the mood for it. Distraction-free is good: you don't need the faff of answering phones when you're slippery, and if the thought makes you smile you're heading in the right direction: away from stresses, towards life force. You're basting yourself, making your skin and then muscles relax with every stroke you make.

Head and neck are great places to start, since as a society we've put far too much pressure on what happens inside the skull and gets there through eyes and ears. A (small) wine glass of oil is about the right amount and dip your fingertips into it to know the feeling before anointing yourself. Yes, anoint. You are divine.

Using the substance of your hand rather than fingers, enjoy working the oil into your scalp and face. Avoid where it could get into eyes, ears, mouth, or nose – there's plenty of space left to work the oil in and when you're done there go onto your neck. Take time. There's a lot going on within your neck, granted the task of holding a cranium containing the electric jelly that is your brain and connecting it to the spine which will in turn play a major part in ensuring your body does more or less what you'd like it to.

Whatever time you have available for self-massage, a good rule of thumb is to devote half of it to your head and neck. For the rest, apply oil to every part you'll be working with, giving it the chance to start doing its work while you're doing the neck-up work. Go for your arms next, leaving the hands until last so you can focus on below the shoulder and then beneath the elbow. Use slow circular motions and inhabit those sensations as you do.

Chest is the next area to treat, remembering to be gentle in your movements – circular always - around the heart. Be similarly sensitive as you progress down to the abdomen, paying attention to and following the way your bowel works – it starts on the right, works its way down left.

After that, your back may be feeling left out, so be sure to do what you can to work with the areas available to reach. Imagine giving yourself a loving hug to make your hands reach that little bit further to spread the love.

Finally, give your legs the same kind of treat as your arms experienced, and using the same principle: hips to knees first, then knees to ankles. And save the best for last. Your feet deserve a special treat for carrying you around all day and all your life, so be sure to lavish special attention on them...almost as much as you'd give to your head.

If you feel moved to thank your body parts for what they're doing, or spend extra time on some areas, go with those instincts. For now at least you're a bit more divine than usual even, and can and should worship and adore yourself. Learning more about the technicalities and fine details of massage and oils and the rest can wait for another time. If you're not approaching it with the right attitude, you're not doing it right. That attitude starts with the heart. Everything and anything else is detail.

MASSAGE AS HEALING

You don't need to be a champion athlete, or even a sports lover, to benefit from the ability of massage that works with muscle and connective tissue and shapes not just your bodily habits, but patterns of thoughts and emotion. For such transformative massage to take effect, it needs to get deep into your body, which requires time. First, outer muscles need to be relaxed – repeated stretches and breathing can be vital in this phase. Only when that's been achieved can deeper musculature be reached. That exploration may also affect tendons and ligaments, with blood vessels and oxygenation too affected, all of which can then lead to changes in the skeletal system. That's the kind of subtle and powerful work that will release older patterns – of breathing, of posture, of reflex – and allow newer ones to emerge, reflecting the world now and not the environment and contexts where those former habits were acquired.

Such patterns can also be about more than our personal history. They can clearly have emotional and psychological importance, and some hold that they are spiritually significant too. You don't have to believe that to get benefit from a skilled massage by a sensitive Ayurvedic practitioner, but in the Vedic tradition among others it's held that memories of previous lives can be something we carry that is a possible limitation. Thinking back to my own experience on the Ealing sofa that connected me to ancient sages in the Himalayas, I'm open to the idea. And remember, the concept of epigenetic stress now being accepted in mainstream science dovetails with that notion of inheritance shaping our bodies, our minds, our sense of who we are and our possibilities.

And there's always Cher of course. *If I Could Turn Back Time*, she sang. She was right. A damn good massage is one way to do it, and return renewed and revitalized, if not quite resurrected.

For dosha specific oils see www.tri-dosha.co.uk

IT'S YOUR TURN

Think of some times when physical expression or exertion has been a meaningful experience for you.

It could have been a time when an outdoor excursion on foot or by bike led you to see not just an amazing view but consider yourself in a new light.

Maybe recovering from an operation taught you about living with limitations or moving beyond them.

A special sexual experience that was both more than physical and intimate in new ways could have had a spiritual aspect.

Did dancing into the small hours create a sense of a identify beyond the personal?

Consider such experiences, what they tell you about yourself, losing that sense of self, and their lingering effect when normality returns. As you do so, move in ways that help heighten the memory. Maybe wear clothes or play music or look at images associated with that time. You might be self-conscious at first. Go with it. Allow your body to guide you.

...AND BREATHE

PANCHAKARMA

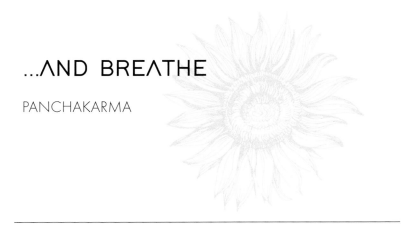

Put bluntly, there are times in our lives when we're full of it. To be fair we're not entirely responsible. The conflicting messages about how to be a person that we acquire from family and friends, from advertising and the media, from education and employers, are a lot to take on. Integrating them into something which makes sense isn't easy. Especially when we become aware of paradoxes, inconsistencies, and hypocrisies that aren't often spoken about and affect the way we take in and respond to the world.

Ever speculated with colleagues that your boss is a sociopath or psychopath? It took a recent report by researchers at the University of Maryland to confirm a primary reason some companies choose one senior management candidate over others is their willingness to transgress ethical boundaries. Which also means someone further up the food chain chose them for that reason, and they in turn were hired with that outcome in mind. See *Recruiting Dark Personalities for Earnings Management* by Ling L. Harris, Scott B. Jackson, Joel Owens, and Nicholas Seybert in the Journal of Business Ethics, May 2021.

It's reasonable to assume things go that way straight to the top, which would explain a lot about the state of the world. Somewhere inside us, we have an awareness of how wrong things are, and that life as lived has only a passing relationship to the serving suggestions we've seen on shows like Friends or in romcoms. We feel the difference with family members when half of what's meant to be a special day together is taken with people being on their phones, ourselves included. If not then, in the realisation we may be living with our parents for years to come at an age we assumed we'd have a home of our own. In groups of friends where more and more are suffering allergies that didn't seem to exist a couple of decades ago. In understanding we don't want to bring children into this world.

All of 'that'...a profound cognitive and emotional load to carry day to day, has potential to create trauma in various forms. However well you look after yourself, and whatever means you have for doing so, it's not surprising so many are overstressed, unbalanced, or otherwise out of sorts with the person you know we can be on even a normal day, never mind a good one. Being otherwise would be the bigger surprise. You've probably noticed it in yourself. Alternately, fingers crossed someone who cares found a way to let you know without your demonstrating just how right their diagnosis is by exploding at them or collapsing into quaking bipedal jelly.

If it's an accessible option for you, then having a few days to give body-mind a thorough detox and work through the physical, mental, emotional, and spiritual matters creating that low is thoroughly recommended. Panchakarma is the name for the Ayurvedic take on an experience that other cultures address through (for example) sweat lodges or ayahuasca journeys. All are rituals of deep personal regeneration for when you deep down know a week on a beach or golf course just won't cut it.

YOU GET TO LIGHT THROUGH WHAT'S HEAVY AND DARK

Panchakarma isn't something to experience lightly. Lightness of movement, of thought, of perceptions and feelings and soul may be the result. But the processes involved in achieving that will necessarily be unsettling at times. What else? You'll be disposing of toxins and whatever else you just don't need any more, and in doing so realising the ways your physiology has adapted to carrying surplus baggage of every sort and becoming aware of the consequences all of that has had for the person you are.

Such a purging experience is a lot to go through purely in its physicality. But body is mind is soul, something we need reminding every time to chip away at the con it could be otherwise. Meaning that panchakarma is a very embodied way of dealing with what psychologists of a Jungian persuasion would call the shadow. What lurks in the shadows? Those things we imagine but don't actually see. They're aspects of yourself you'd rather not dwell on though might over time have come to appreciate are doing something useful even if you'd prefer to be ignorant of the precise what and how and why.

Put coarsely then panchakarma is literally about sorting your shit out. And that involves accepting shit is no more or less than a byproduct of what you eat. Anything else in your response is an unnecessary complication introduced by thought or feeling as they relate to some or other combination of upbringing, childhood memories, and reading too much Freud about all of those and what they 'mean'. Trust me, poo doesn't mean, though it can smell that way.

Panchakarma is more than a healthcare procedure, it's a rite of passage lasting several days. That function is especially important in a culture that's largely put ritual and ceremony to one side except for when they present opportunities to make money or display power. Even in modern India it's something fewer are finding time for, let alone going through it thrice yearly as the sages recommend. But panchakarma remains something that keeps at least some of the elite on their feet. It's not an indulgence.

ITERATION IS INTEGRATION (ALSO, PIANOS)

If you learn to play piano, you'll get presented with a keyboard that has 49 or 61 or 88 keys. So many notes! So much to learn! Except it isn't. It just looks that way. In practice there are just 12 different notes. Really. It's just that they repeat.

Here's how it works. You know the black notes? They're divided into a group of three, and a pair. To the left of the first in a pair, that white key is a C. With a full 88 keys there are 11 of those runs of notes, each with a C. Yes, they are lower at one end and higher at the other. But they're recognisably the same sound.

It takes a while to get used to all this. Running your fingers up and down the white notes, discovering the different sound possibilities when you mix white and black keys in one 11-note group. Then seeing what happens when you explore playing the same tune over a bigger stretch of the piano.

Get good at that, and you might get a certificate letting the world know you're Grade 8. And maybe take it further still – joining an orchestra to play established works or getting into the improvisatory possibilities of jazz. But still, you're dealing with just the same notes. Only now you're not just more technically capable – you have insights now that weren't available to you as a novice.

In doing all this, your hearing has changed. The music you hear as you go about the world you may be able to transpose onto keyboards without even looking for the score or making notation. Birdsong, the ebb and flow of conversation, light between the branches of a tree in the garden, all can become the basis of new music, able to enter the world though your fingers in the form of a tune that never existed before, even though millions of musicians have played the piano for centuries.

Those initial tentative attempts to play Chopsticks (seemingly a given whenever you start) become, depending on your age and preferences, your own take on Prince or Madonna, Beethoven or Bruce Springsteen. And a few will perform on stage, sharing with audiences their love of Mozart or providing backing for Cher.

As with keyboard skills, so with Ayurveda.

The basics are everything. And they aren't remotely basic. They're the stuff of life itself. Skin and muscle and breath and thought and posture and nutrition and exercise are fundamentals that you will be learning more about across your life even if you don't notice you're paying attention.

It's that gradual development of learning that allows you to sense that hint of kapha in a client you'd thought was vata. The shift of season that you interpret with new pitta energy before the word has formed in your mind. The awareness that a different oil would be better than the sesame you initially had in mind before the client comes in for a massage and you hear the story their skin tells.

Everything you ever need to know about how to respond to someone you're working with ayurvedically is there when they come through the door. It might not all be apparent that instant, or in your early years of practice, but over time your ability to respond to information that was previously invisible to you, and to ask the right questions when they count, will ensure that your skills and understanding develop, and with them your awareness that there is always more to discover. And the understanding is there...somewhere.

The core of Ayurveda is that the universe is fundamentally simple but arranged by humans to be inordinately complex. We're encouraged to stick with and to that complexity, but it really won't help. Staying with that focus on deep and rich simplicity is what allows solutions to emerge. And that's what makes the experience of panchakarma the experience of a multi-day Rachmaninov recital for an audience of one – the client lucky enough to receive that treatment.

WHY PANCHAKARMA TAKES SEVERAL DAYS

Given panchakarma is in effect a process of rebirth, it's not surprising that it takes a long time. Especially in a culture where people experience stresses of sorts that didn't exist centuries ago thanks to their jobs and the condition of the environment. And a society that for the most part treats wellbeing as a way of keeping more workers productive for longer, rather than as a birthright, inflicts a lot of harm from or even prior to birth, way before the people in need of panchakarma have ever come across Ayurveda.

The process happens across several days and in a number of phases (panchakarma meaning five actions):

1.   *Shamana* – before embarking on panchakarma, ensure you eat a light and healthy diet for a week beforehand. Rice and vegetables and lentils recommended, meat and dairy are off the menu. Daily exercise is also part of shamana.

2.   *Purvakarma* is the initial step in panchakarma. You first go through *2a. snehana*, which includes a massage of herb-infused oils specific to you as an individual in line with your dosha and medical history. The purpose is in part to soothe or stimulate you according to your profile and response in the moment, and to get a greater sense of the impact of diet on your current state.

Eating lots of processed food for many years can affect energy levels thanks to running on poor quality nutrients that don't support a robust immune system. There can be mental and emotional effects too. So in the snehana period you'll also ingest a fatty substance – either snehana itself or *ghee* (clarified butter).

Thanks to them your body will gradually release *ama* (toxins) during the course of the treatment. Each is a healthy option compared to many of the fats you'll have ingested deep into your tissues, and those malefactors will pretty much glom onto or gloop with the snehana or ghee. *2b. Svedana* – part sauna and part steam bath, the intent here is to embark on a deep cleanse, inside and out. Sweating out toxins that massage brings to the surface goes along with the impact of the snehana to ready you for...

3.   *Virechana*. You're already on your way to an experience of purging which a mild mix of oil and herbs is well placed to accelerate, ensuring that by the time you make use of the toilet your frequent visits will feel as gentle and liberating as can be. Ginger tea will be on standby to soothe any unpleasant sensations.

With bowels clear, and a rising sense of revitalisation, it's time for light meals as per the shamana rice and veggie and lentil diet. Chamomile or licorice tea are good as part of an overall relaxed atmosphere, and you're making progress on a path away from headaches, skin conditions, and other stress-related phenomena.

4.   *Basti*. The western equivalent is enemas, in this case one oil-based and the other water-based. Unlike most enemas as they're understood in the west, these involve the ingestion of herbal preparations to introduce potent healing agents internally. And the general reckoning is they account for half the effectiveness of the panchakarma journey.

5.   *Rasayana* – this is all about going back into the world healed and staying that way. Panchakarma is not something to be experienced lightly, and rasayana is about the art of longevity as practiced in part through making better dietary choices.

AND BACK AGAIN

Why the emphasis on foods? Simply put, we are what we eat. And western diet choices tend to be based on marketing and convenience, neither of which tends to lead to healthy nutrition. Packaging emphasises colours and shapes to trigger responses that have no connection to what's within the box or tin or sachet. Brand is all, and even when – as with Cadbury's say – the company is bought by an American corporation and the quality of the chocolate (never brilliant to begin with) goes downhill, the familiar purple wrappers entice shoppers seeking a quick hit of fats and sugars.

Those substances are the building blocks for...us. A reminder of the seven tissues which we're made of:

Rasa – lymph/plasma

Rakta – blood

Mamsa – muscle

Medas – fat

Asthi – bone

Majja – marrow/nerve

Shukra – reproductive organs

That substance – which makes us, us – is comprised in large part of the stuff in your cupboards, fridge, or bin. No judging - but have a look and see if you'd be happy to make a person out of them. None of this prevents us enjoying the occasional pizza or ice cream, but next time you hear someone say in a kind of patronising way that an older person is looking well-preserved, it might just be food preservatives they're seeing.

Ayurveda aims higher. We are beings that exist in different dimensions while being anchored to this one. Tapping into our personal power requires us to restore the strength of Agni (digestive fire) and its balance with Ojas (which fuels spiritual growth). And doing so calls for focus. Not the endless distraction of this week's diet or the latest faddish ingredient but using the principles of Ayurveda to make better choices in the physical and consumer environment you find yourself.

Another piano metaphor might be helpful. American jazz player Paul Bley said of the instrument, that of its 88 keys there are just a handful of good ones. Ayurveda is all about steering a path aligned with core concepts stretching back millennia. Bearing those principles in mind will steer you better around food than stepping into a supermarket and allowing your nervous system to be hijacked by the chirpy instore radio station, strategically-positioned attention-grabbing merchandise stands that companies pay lots for because they know shoppers gravitate to them, and shelves whose contents are based less on your needs than research showing what's most profitable.

The underlying message of such consumer emporiums, where we hungry ghosts push trolleys and never quite seem to get what we came for however hard we try, is that plenty is an illusion. The brightly lit aisles are more about sensory stimulation to keep us in a permanent state of novelty on steroids.

If you doubt that based on your experience of shopping for food at the local Tesco, consider instead your response to IKEA. When did you lose your IKEA virginity? Was it good for you? What the furniture-to-meatballs store did brilliantly was combine supermarket thinking with design skills from theatre and film...not for the furniture itself, but in the creation of small sets where it's easy to imagine hanging out with family and friends. It takes an active choice to look up and realise you're walking in is, practically speaking, an aircraft hangar.

As with IKEA, so the world in general some of the time. Being made constantly on edge by the demands of work, the treadmill of productivity, the apparent need to compete is hard. The capacity to connect with family and friends in meaningful ways is drained by that expenditure of energy, leaving many of us exhausted and increasingly so.

IT'S YOUR TURN

Get a notebook and sit down with that and a pen and a drink of something soothing and non-alcoholic. Start to think back over the last week, and review experiences that you can list on separate pages under these headings:

Good Intentions

Here, list times you set out to make good choices and got things done but didn't quite make things happen how you hoped. There are probably good reasons for that, and this isn't about judging, more about noticing yourself with compassion.

Losing It

In this section, record instances where things just…didn't work, for whatever reason at all or none that you have insight into. Mornings you ended up at a café not a gym. Evenings spent watching Ally McBeal boxsets instead of meditating and applying for a new job. Arguments with neighbours.

Coping

How do you handle stresses, anxieties, perceived failures? Are you a secret smoker? Problem drinker? Have KFC on automatic dial? Resort to a lover you know is bad news but provides comfort for a few hours? The ways we punish ourselves with rewards that can harm us are worth looking at rather than experiencing shame about.

You could keep these lists for a while, adding to them to get a better picture over a few weeks or months. And just having them on paper will help give you more sense of who you are and where your flashpoints can be found.

Looking at what comes up, see what emerges as you let yourself consider small simple changes. Maybe 15 minutes of yoga before work every day rather than aiming for a one hour class a couple of times a week. Wandering round Tesco reciting or listening to a mantra to see if it results in different items in your basket. Being firm about no fried breakfast for you when you visit your parents at the weekend if it leaves you feeling depleted all day.

Stick to the basics – there's nothing else

The starting premise of Ayurveda is that the universe has only a few core aspects and a myriad ways to experience them. Society has evolved to offer the illusion of choice in the form of an impossible number of consumer offerings, geared not for your benefit but for that of the businesses presenting them. Which they do relentlessly, on every screen imaginable. And those businesses do not have your best interests at heart. Especially the interests of your heart itself.

Every choice we make is a footprint that takes us one way or another. The habitual path we've made is the easiest to follow, by definition. But in doing so, especially at this point in history when the world is notably crazy, we put ourselves at risk. Doing what we're used to is the essence of homeostasis, which is to do with maintaining our systems as they are since changing them expends energy in the hope of acquiring more – which is a risk.

To make more sense of that, think back to earlier times. You lived in a village with a few other families, growing a few crops. A few people would go into woods to hunt and come back with a boar, say. The risk of not finding a boar or being injured by one was there, but the village would get by thanks to the vegetables being grown, and preserved or stored foods such as pickles and cheese.

If you want to leave that village, curious about going downriver by canoe to visit a town you've heard about, you're taking a risk for sure. Both for yourself, and in removing your capacity to provide (and much more besides) from the village. You'll be leaving the networks of people and place that have sustained you. But in the town you may be able to learn new skills, and through trading what you know from village life return there one day and integrate your greater understandings in the context of the community you grew up.

As with villages, so with individuals. The many aspects that make us up are ones we can get greater insight into thanks to the core concepts of Ayurveda. If you recognise the need to make a course correction to become more of the person you know in your bones you're capable of becoming, the knowledge is there. And how you nourish yourself is at the core. What you take in, as food and drink, as entertainment and information, as emotion and thought, is something we can change. And the tools for doing so are all there in the fundamentally simple approach enshrined in this ancient approach to life. You might not have the time or resources to do a fullblown panchakarma at this point and may never have. But the principles and practices involved are ones that can be incorporated into your daily life, starting right now – before you begin the final chapter. Wouldn't it be great to get a head start on the rest of this incarnation before the end of this book?

BREAKING POINT

SPIRITUALITY AND THE FUTURE

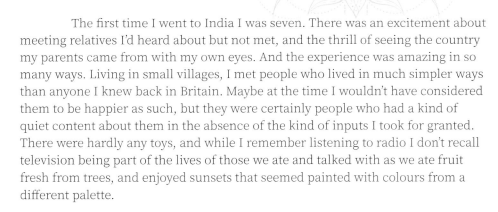

The first time I went to India I was seven. There was an excitement about meeting relatives I'd heard about but not met, and the thrill of seeing the country my parents came from with my own eyes. And the experience was amazing in so many ways. Living in small villages, I met people who lived in much simpler ways than anyone I knew back in Britain. Maybe at the time I wouldn't have considered them to be happier as such, but they were certainly people who had a kind of quiet content about them in the absence of the kind of inputs I took for granted. There were hardly any toys, and while I remember listening to radio I don't recall television being part of the lives of those we ate and talked with as we ate fruit fresh from trees, and enjoyed sunsets that seemed painted with colours from a different palette.

Years later, as a business journalist, I lived in nine countries in the bubble of luxury hotel life. More accurately it feels sometimes that I lived in just one generically exclusive hotel which magically changed location, and I'd only know where for sure because the local language and cuisine were different once you got out into the streets. I met hundreds of CEOs and managing directors and company founders, and every now and then I spoke with one who had a flicker of vision, of hope for something other than a more profitable year. In Egypt I was fascinated for a while by pictures of President Mubarak that everyone had in their offices and homes. Clearly a man whose values and example inspired his people. Then I learned people were obliged to have his image on display and potentially face penalties if they didn't.

The third time I visited India, in 2002, things were very different. Hoping to reconnect with the country I'd come to love, this time round - working for the press agency - I was soon sick to my soul. The CEOs I met were glamoured by rising graphs and lowering costs just the same as any others I'd encountered. And they lived in superficially impressive homes. An overdose of glitz on every wall – and somewhere in a basement, servants who were effectively slaves living in grim conditions.

The deep wrongness of it all is what catalysed my breakdown. It transformed me, allowed me through Ayurveda to discover the person I always was in some way, and am, and will be as I continue to shed the labels and limits that contain me for a while, before they too constrain me and allow another Sunita to emerge.
Is this the world we created?

Whether you want to apply the world spirituality to the conversation or not, the fact that our world is at crisis point thanks to the determination of a tiny number of people with incalculable wealth and power to accumulate more of both is an unprecedented obscenity. The amount of effort put into keeping humans worldwide at each other's throats on social media and in the streets is indicative of the fear underlying their determination to control.

One group of people who you won't come across on social media are children mining rare earth minerals required for use in our telephones, and the ever-proliferating digital nodules in your house under the banner IOT. The initials stand for Internet of Things, and the things in question are thermostats, washing machines, televisions, and more, all with their usage monitored in tiny detail. It's true that such data can be used to provide efficiencies, but only if you look within the very limited frame you're invited to as a consumer.

That idea of illth mentioned before – of the bad consequences unacknowledged in the creation of wealth – is sickeningly apparent when you look at the costs involved in rare earth minerals.

They are mined in dismal conditions. 60% to 70% of the world's cobalt, used in renewables such as car batteries and phones, is found in the Democratic

Republic of Congo. There it is extracted by around 35,000 children as young as five. Their lives are a living hell – it's not just incredibly dangerous, but many lose limbs or are raped by those who supervise them.

Among the companies using Congolese cobalt are Apple, Tesla, Microsoft, and Google. Other rare earth suppliers are available – not least because Afghanistan has potentially $3 trillion worth of them. Both America and China are very interested in getting access to those minerals, which has alarming implications for continued geopolitical struggle in that country.

The extraction process involved to mine the minerals also results in radioactive waste. And nobody knows what to do with it other than store it somewhere a long way away. In Malaysia the Lynas Advanced Materials Plant amassed over 1.5 million tonnes of waste between 2011 and 2018, about a third of it radioactive. Some of the waste is also toxic to the area's groundwater. In February 2020 the company was ordered to build a permanent disposal facility, the deadline for which has been extended to March 2022 because of Covid.

MEANWHILE IN MIDDLE-EARTH

Italian pastry chef Nicolas Gentile owns a small piece of land in Italy where he lives with his family in a house built to resemble a home that a hobbit from *Lord of the Rings* could live in. Tolkien's stories have been a lifelong inspiration for Nicola, but this is far from a form of escapism he said in an interview with *The Guardian*. "I am living my dream, my adventure. By purchasing that piece of land, I have removed it from a reality that I don't like and am shaping it the way I want."

Already the area chosen has a celebration called Banderesi where people dress and prepare dishes as they have for centuries, and even outside the festival Gentile says people in the area live like hobbits. By this he means they are close to nature. And, like the hobbits in the books and films, he took a ring on a long journey to a volcano – Mount Vesuvius.

The canoli maker's dream is of creating a village with solar powered homes, and the response he had from strangers on his long quest convinced him of its possibility. People welcomed him into their homes, fed him and let him stay overnight, compelled by what he was doing. He sees their reaction as magical.

Rewind over a century, and Tolkien experienced visions, initially between 1911 and 1913, that led him to draw images of mythic places and creatures. Dragons, caves, mountains. This work became the foundation of what he called *The Red Book of Westmarch*, that came to include the stories that made Tolkien's name known worldwide.

Also in 1913, the psychologist Carl Jung began his Red Book, an outpouring of images and words that was to form the basis of his life's work. The parallels in subject of artwork and theme are uncanny, as elaborated in an extraordinary PhD thesis by astrologer Becca Tarnas. Both men were sure what they had found – or found them – was in some ways a response to a planet experiencing its first World War, which Tolkien fought in. And Jung was sure his act of unexpected and sometimes terrifying creativity was far from escapism. "To give birth to the ancient in a new time is creation...The task is to give birth to the old in a new time."

That need is even more urgent now, and Italian pastry chef's example – untutored by reading of Jung but driven in exactly the way he described – is one of many at this point. We need them. And Jung himself? He was writing what he knew. This was a man who carved rocks he quarried and made a tower of them in which he created the Red Book.

THE STAKES ARE HIGH

On one hand we have Tolkien's pint-sized heroes, elven archers, and in Gandalf a wizard who'd be equally at home in Jung's world of cosmic forces. On the other we have...*Pokemon* Go. At any rate, the cartoon characters you or kids in your life may have wanted to collect at some point took on a new form of existence when the Japanese animated characters became the basis of a whole new kind of entertainment.

It looked like harmless fun on the surface at least: people discovering the cute critturs using their phones in parks, on buildings, in an international extravaganza that gave hints about the way things are going. Augmented and virtual reality are part of that, with digital leisure activities around every corner as businesses find new ways to make money in the imaginal realm.

Pokemon Go was also an experiment in discovering what it takes for people to behave in new ways with a pretty much imaginary incentive. The business who created the game - Niantic Labs – was founded by John Hanke, also CEO of mapping company Keyhole Inc (responsible for Google Earth), funded by the CIA's venture capital branch, In-Q-Tel. Their webpage is upfront:

"Visionary startups. Experienced VCs. Dedicated government professionals. In-Q-Tel leads from the center of this matrix, connecting cutting-edge technology, strategic investments, and purpose: to enhance and advance national security for the U.S. and its allies."

You can take for granted that the game hoovered up an eyebrow-raising amount of data from players. Among the numerous people credited for *Pokemon* Go, the names of Congolese children whose miserable existences make it possible for the game to be played are not included.

While it's undeniably true that things really are dismal in so many ways at a macro level right now, taking that on board every moment is not the way we get through it. And never has been. There's pretty much always an earthquake happening somewhere while your family gets good news. Lottery wins and cancer diagnoses sometimes coincide. Each is for sure part of a bigger tapestry, but how we react is a matter of choice. And choice starts with connecting who we are in a moment that resonates not just the here and now but with eternity.

It's in eternity where we start, where we always have been, and are, and forever will be. But that's at the level of *Atman*, far beyond consciousness in any way we can usefully appreciate except when we get fleeting glimpses in moments of bliss and joy. Between those precious jewels on the necklace of the cosmos are threaded job interviews and bad dates and Netflix and car repairs and new school uniforms and Zoom meetings always Zoom meetings and did you speak to the vet and sourdough bloody sourdough and maybe a week in a Welsh cottage and washing machine expiring just out of warranty and lifedrawing classes and funeral arrangements and today's the optician and this slowcooker really is slow and bloaty stomach and snagged toenail again and lost headphones and wasted gym membership and too many jigsaw pieces and bad wallpaper moments and juicing and awkward mask conversations and retirement homes and hayfever and red cabbage coleslaw and latest gossip and Amazon deliveries and Elon Musk and essential oil sprays and superhero movies and garage sales and diabetes checks and charity shop raffles and chicken quarters and new phone contracts and sun-hats and asthma inhalers and cheese dilemmas and batik and candle crises and and and and and and.

AYURVEDA CHARTS THE SACRED

All of which is why, given the sheer amount of everything there is, it helps to have something to put it all in and navigate around as best you can. And that's pretty much the **why** of Ayurveda. Look at it as a map to connect us with moments of the sacred and make it possible to encounter more of them more frequently and more powerfully along our way. We do so using tools that are our inheritance as sentient beings: bodies that allow us to move through the material world, senses through which we make it known to us, and a mind allowing us to make choices. Only, the same tools can take us to misery and worse, so...choose wisely.

Ayurveda's maps are contained in texts known as **Upanishads**. The name sounds rather grand until you discover some translate it along the lines of 'sit down close'. Which would be like calling *The Bible,* 'pull up a chair'. It's friendly, welcoming. Has a touch of *Hitch-Hiker's Guide To The Galaxy* about it even.

A key part of what makes maps of use is that their ability to describe features we recognise and help us identify those we don't. Start at Derby, take the motorway, and you'll get to Sheffield. That kind of thing. Only, with maps of sacred states, many many people will either deny the existence of such destinations or dismiss them by saying that they were - for instance - merely the result of being with a particular group of people on a great night where everyone had a good time. You may know how it goes, almost like a head teacher giving a talk to the school:

"We all made it to Blackpool for an end of term event. Most of us were satisfied with a night where the mood was set by music and moonlight and mirth. (*Significant pause, eyebrow raised.*) But that's not enough for everyone is it? A few oddballs decided that wasn't enough and what they experienced was divinity."

So be it.

If you do accept the utility of a framework that will allow you to revisit some of that sacred territory again, odds are you'll find that it can do so. And it comes with a price…return visits won't ever quite be the same.

Going back can become like trying to tickle yourself, which simply can't be done. Or rather, the tickling can be, but no way will it come with the response that happens when somebody else does it. Atman can be similarly tricky, but fortunately manifests in many forms. A spectacular sunset. A phone call from the right person at the right time. A passage in a book. A spoonful of perfectly chilled strawberry yoghurt.

If we're a microcosm of the cosmos, then what could be mapped but us? Or at any rate, notes made by previous passengers on Spaceship Earth as they add their observations to the wisdom of former visitors. A key one, drawn from millennia of observations of what it's like to be our kind of biped, is that what we consider mind can be said to have four different aspects:

Manas – the sensory or processing mind, which takes in information gathered through the senses and arranges it in ways that makes most sense to the perceiver at any given moment. That allows manas to alert you to an oncoming motorbike when you really don't need the possible hospital trip, though won't make the decision of what to do with that information.

Ahamkara – this is what we know as I. Which often gets a bad press in the west as ego. Given that we're small creatures on an enormous planet where there is peril of every sort not far away, having a healthy sense of who we are, what we aren't, and that we're worth looking after is a good thing. Not least because who would care for those who matter to us in our absence?

Citta – those things which take our attention in life can be viewed as themes and are experienced emotionally. They're as likely to crop up around people and places as colours and tastes and play an important part in shaping perceptions – usefully at times, and less so as well. Some say that they're shaped by past life experiences.

Buddhi – our consciousness, which takes the sensory material we're presented with and incorporates it into a form that allows us to make decisions. It may be the case we won't know what the basis of those choices is, save when we reflect on our lives over time, and spot what we've been drawn to or repelled from.

All of this is good, and there are analogies in Western psychology. And already, within this conception it's possible to see the individual as a body riding in a chariot pulled by horses, on its way to a destination. Problem being, the environment that chariot is travelling through. Those horses need sustenance in the form of food and water. Rest, too. And they deserve a treat, surely. Which can easily shift from being something that offers nourishment and reward and instead puts horses and rider into a rajasic carb coma...

It's tricky managing bodymind in a consumer society that encourages overwork and overstimulates us with caffeine and digital stimuli to present the appearance of energy. With growing knowledge of how the microbiome works we can take a more sophisticated approach to nourishment allied with the wealth of Ayurvedic knowledge contained within dosha lore.

All of that is good and allows us to steer a clearer path. But there's an underlying problem. Consumer culture wants nothing more from people than their money and loyalty, and it will stop at pretty much nothing to acquire customers for life. Such an outlook is only possible within a materialist worldview with no sense that there's a cosmology beyond the bottom line. If you doubt that, ask yourself how we end up in a situation where senior oil company employees were duped in 2021 by a Greenpeace journalist poising as a recruitment consultant. The high-flyers outlined PR strategies they use to give the appearance of being environmentally-friendly while in practice stalling change even further, allowing their employer Exxon to keep profiting from the knowing destruction of the one and only planet that's our home.

Advertising, marketing, and social media are all about pressing buttons for fear and shame and suggesting they can be papered over with the purchase of whatever product is being pimped that second. And it has to be this second right now – another part of the brain chemistry game being played is the recognition Fear of Missing Out can be a motivator.

MAINSTREAM HEALTH SYSTEMS ARE FAIING US

The unmerry-go-round of overstimulation is a soul-destroying one. But in a culture that doesn't recognise soul it's instead an excuse for prescription in some form. Being numb feels pretty attractive some days and helps explain why the Sackler family got away with selling opioids under the name OxyContin from their company Purdue Pharma that killed 600,000 Americans. The legal deal they came to means they are immune from further civil suits about the matter and will soon be even wealthier billionaires than they already were. In Purdue's efforts to defend OxyContin, Dr Richard Sackler claimed any overdoses that occurred were the responsibility of "criminal addicts".

What's happening in the NHS at this point also has worrying aspects as American-style approaches get more of a hold. There's no doubt that the NHS and its component services are massively stretched because of covid, which – directly and indirectly - has had a huge impact on mental health countrywide.

A friend I'll call Beth worked as a Psychological Wellbeing Practitioner within the Talking Therapies Service, itself part of Improved Access To Psychological Therapies. She only lasted a few months. Beth's role was to recommend basic Cognitive Behavioural Therapy (CBT) techniques contained within booklets.

CBT has its place, but this was surface level stuff that could only scratch the surface of what was happening for people now. For many, bigger and older issues were being brought up by the experience of pandemic which CBT was ill-equipped for. Clients were asked to fill in a PHQ9 form to score nine questions about their depression, and a GAD7 to rate their experience of generalised anxiety disorder.

As a Patient Wellbeing Practitioner, Beth had to interview, assess, and complete documentation in 100 minutes total for two patients daily to a rigid timetable. Which is itself problematic: not only can mental health problems be reduced to a score of 1-9 or 1-7, they also require paperwork done to inform the patient's GP.

The remainder of Beth's day would be taken up doing 30-minute sessions with clients whose scores made them eligible for support. At any rate, for six weeks: Beth and her colleagues were encouraged to accentuate the positive so that their work can be completed in that period and new patients taken on. It's not a therapeutic model, it's a business model. See those scores drop, Beth and the system are clearly doing a great job, contract renewed.

But such cookie-cutter approaches have an effect. We're not made of cookie dough, and nothing in this approach takes account of the PWP's own mental health, which having listened to 7 people daily and being incentivised with ongoing career prospects to maintain is itself likely to suffer. It probably works for some people, and that's fine. But structurally that's a by-product rather than a feature of what's going on.

Maybe Beth's experience is just a one-off? I don't think so. And others concur. The NHS was noted as providing the world's best healthcare by the Commonwealth Fund in 2014 and 2017. By 2021 we ranked ninth in the world for healthcare outcomes – ie the ability of patients to recover after the treatment they received. The fact we'd also dropped to fourth place for accessibility of care and the admin systems involved, and fifth for the processes used in care, probably helps explain that slump.

AND THERE IS HOPE

We cannot rely on current models of how the world should be to give us the kind of life we need to thrive. And by thrive I don't simply mean economic abundance. Our current patterns of consumption are toxic. Thriving in the sense of fruition, and both words pointing to a more organic and freer version of existence.

There's a fundamental sickness to societies and economies trapped in a model where self-worth and status are both achieved through purchasing power, and the money to pay for it all is earned by working too long for businesses that typically have no concern for anything beyond the bottom line. It nearly destroyed me in my journalistic career, and if OxyContin isn't a clear demonstration of just how irrevocably fucked things can be I don't know what is.

Whatever we do it needs to be done to a different tune than the ones we hear on Spotify to blank out any inconvenient thoughts and feelings as we embark on another day in another year in another millennium on a planet that has seen civilizations come and go and is itself part of a solar system orbiting a sun which is responsible for life in all forms and all of us connected in a dance with billions of other stars in an unfathomably vast cosmos which has rhythms infinitely more complex and joyous than even the most elegantly assembled spreadsheet.

We don't have to live our lives nudged about by anxieties orchestrated by cynical use of social media data that will never satisfy us beyond the short term buzz a new pair of shoes or pizza or car can provide. Ayurveda points to a living cosmos that we are woven into and always have been. It exists in the form of *Purusha*, which you can think of as more male and to do with soul and self and consciousness. And it can be found in *Prakuti*, which can be considered more female, and concerns substance and nature and source.

The constant engagement and flow of Prakuti and Purusha as they unfold is what forms the unseen and intangible backdrop to our lives and the universe itself. Our own awareness of it is possible thanks to *Mahat*, which contains all the other descriptions of consciousness and mind that apply within Ayurveda, that we looked at earlier: Manas, Ahamkara, Cittas, and Buddhi.

Really, the names are just that. But so are the names of our friends, and in the same way we can like and love and be frustrated by our friends, so too can we by our experience of mind. And we know too that when all is flowing, that those names matter not at all, and that the joy of a moment that might be something we can find in every moment is what matters more than any of the detritus of life on a planet which to some of its inhabitants is still not long past the teenage years of the 21st century.

And maybe that's a useful way to take it all in. I'm writing this in the 21st year or the 21st century. And 21 is notable in a couple of ways. For a start, it's the number that we're acknowledged as adults in a bigger way than we were at 18, the previous threshold year. At 21 you can apply to adopt a child, stand for election as MP, and hold a licence to fly an aeroplane, helicopter, or gyroplane. So really, it's still early doors on the whole adult thing. But enough years done to know what a good decision feels like and what to steer clear of.

And in many Tarot decks, the 21st card of the Major Arcana (the ones that have the fanciest pictures and names) is The World. It's associated with being male and female, like Prakuti and Purusha. Like any of us, it's between earth and heaven. And it connects us with cosmic consciousness. Ayurveda, as seen through different eyes. And if we are cosmically conscious, then all eyes are one, so how could things be otherwise?

DOSHΛ QUIZ ΛND TΛBLE OF TOOLS

YOUR BODY | MIND TYPE

You'll have seen by now that this Ayurveda book does things differently.

The world doesn't need another ABC guide. There's a place for them, for sure. And Ayurveda is ready for a different kind of book. One that looks back but not in super-massive detail, but instead looks around to present a wider context that Ayurvedic philosophy sits within. Which is why the nods to acupuncture and Gurdjieff, namechecks for Tolkien and Jung, stories about Amazon tribes, eyebrows raised at poor Descartes, and much more besides.

Having been on that mystery tour, you'll have a far greater sense of the concepts and practices which underpin Ayurveda. Which means you're on your way to a broader and deeper and richer comprehension of this millennia-old way of being than when you came in. And in the same way that a visit to the museum ends in the giftshop before returning to the normal world, we'll stop here to do the Dosha Quiz.

Maybe you've done one before. In a magazine, on a website. This time, you'll have more of a sense of the ideas that make doshas useful. And will be aware that your sense of your doshas may change over time, and that different Ayurvedic therapists and practitioners may have a variety of responses to you for reasons that will now be clear. Nobody 'is' a particular dosha. They're colours on a palette which changes with the seasons, and mingle with the other doshas. But enough. Sharpen that pencil. Find that pen. It's time for the dosha quiz!

	VATA	PITTA	KAPHA
Physical body			
Height	☐ Tall or very short	☐ Medium	☐ Usually short, but can be tall and large
Frame	☐ Thin, boney	☐ Moderate, good muscle	☐ Large, well-developed
Weight	☐ Low, difficult to gain	☐ Moderate	☐ Heavy, hard to lose
Skin	☐ Rough, dry, thin	☐ Warm, oily	☐ Cold, oily, thick
Eyes	☐ Small, dry, nervous, often brown	☐ Sharp, penetrating, green, blue or grey with yellowish sclera	☐ Big, beautiful, loving, calm
Hair	☐ Dry, thin, curly	☐ Soft, oily, red, fair	☐ Thick, oily, wavy, lustrous
Nails	☐ Rough, hard, brittle, split easily	☐ Soft, pink, lustrous	☐ Whitish, pale, smooth, polished
Voice	☐ Low or weak, quick - talkative	☐ High or sharp, moderate, clear, precise	☐ Slow, maybe laboured, or deep tonal
Walk	☐ Quick, light, hurried	☐ Medium paced, purposeful	☐ Slow, steady, calm
Physiological			
Common Ailment	☐ nervous, sharp pains, headaches, dry, rash, gas/constipation	☐ inflammation, rashes, allergies, heartburn, ulcers, fevers	☐ fluid retention, excess mucous, ulcers, bronchitis, sinus, asthma
Elimination	☐ Irregular, constipated, hard, dry	☐ Regular, loose	☐ Slow, plentiful and heavy
Sweat	☐ Minimal	☐ profuse, especially when hot	☐ Moderate – but present even when not exercising
Temperature preference	☐ craves warmth, dislikes cold and dry	☐ loves coolness, dislikes heat and sun	☐ Dislikes cold and damp, prefers heat

Category	Option 1	Option 2	Option 3
Appetite	☐ Variable, small	☐ Good, regular	☐ Slow, steady
Digestion	☐ Eat quickly, delicate	☐ Strong, can eat almost anything	☐ Eat and digest slowly
Endurance	☐ Minimal	☐ Moderate	☐ Excellent
Sleep	☐ Poor, disturbed	☐ Moderate but sound	☐ Heavy, prolonged, excessive
Dreams	☐ Frequent, can't remember on waking	☐ vivid, often in colour easy to remember	☐ Only remembers highly significant, clear dreams
Psychological			
Emotions	☐ Enthusiastic, outgoing, changeable ideas and moods	☐ Strong-minded, purposeful, thrives on challenges, express opinion	☐ Calm, placid, good natured, easy going, reliable
Memory	☐ Poor long-term, quick to grasp but forgets	☐ Sharp and clear	☐ Slow to learn but never forgets
Stress	☐ Anxious and nervous	☐ Angry, irritable	☐ Fear and anger if pushed
Work	☐ Quick, imaginative, active and creative thinker, bored with routine	☐ natural leader, efficient, planned routine, perfectionist	☐ keeps things calm, caring, enjoys regular routine
Finances	☐ Poor, spends rapidly	☐ Moderate, buys luxuries	☐ Rich, thrifty
Hobbies	☐ Travel, art, philosophy	☐ Sport, politics, luxuries	☐ Serene, leisurely types
Creativity	☐ Original, fertile	☐ Technical, scientific	☐ Entrepreneurial
Friends	☐ Make and change often	☐ Most work related, change when I change jobs	☐ long lasting and sincere
Lifestyle	☐ Erratic	☐ Busy but plans to achieve much	☐ Steady and regular, maybe stuck in a rut
Total:			

TABLE OF TOOLS

What follows is not definitive. But if you want a quick ready-reckoner for potentially useful things to get you through what's going on with you, then these suggestions arise from decades of my own experience, and the understanding of the Ayurvedic giants whose shoulders I stand on.

VATA

Seasons
Increases in the Autumn.

Foods
Strengthening foods to nourish such as whole grains, lentils and pumpkin. Lemons, tomatoes, yoghurt, cheese which are good for digestion. Butter and ghee are also good for vata, as well as a steady supply of complete proteins in white meat, fresh fish and venison as they build stamina. And warming teas such as ginger and nutmeg which are beneficial in having a carminative effect on this flighty dosha.

Herbs/Spices
For the body - Warming herbs such as ginger, cinnamon, liquorice, ashwagandha, calamus, jatamansi, dashmula.

For cooking – saffron, black pepper, salt, tamari, ajawan, sage, turmeric, rosemary, fennel, cinnamon, bay leaf, cumin, basil.

Movement
Useful yoga asanas (postures) include:

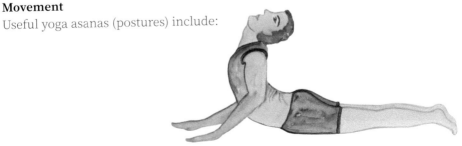

Cobra pose which helps expand the rib cage, chest and abdomen (Figure 1).

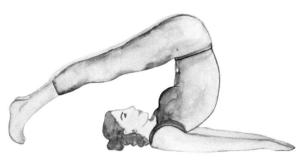

Plow pose which calms the nervous system and reduces stress and fatigue
(Figure 2).

Other exercises: Swimming breast stroke helps ground vata types and strengthens
and opens up the neck, shoulders, and back muscles.

Breath
Alternate nostril breathing helps balance wayward energy and improves brain
function when concentration and clarity is poor.

Massage
Best suited to more flowing rhythmic movements using a soothing oil blend to
calm and relax the body.

PITTA

Seasons
Dominates late Spring (which can set Pitta ailments in motion, eg: hayfever).

Foods
To keep pitta, the fire element, in balance it is best to curtail your intake of spicy
foods during this time, and control the amount of sour, salty and pungent tastes
which are all heat producing such as sour fruits (tomatoes in particular) and
instead favouring foods which are cooling and refreshing including vegetables in
abundance such as asparagus, broccoli, brussels sprouts, sprouts and cabbage,
cooling herbs like fresh coriander and dill, and pulses, however over consumption

of the latter can cause acidity so be careful to eat this in moderation.

Herbs/Spices
For sensitive skin and an aggravated digestive tract, herbs such as neem, shata-vari, amalaki, fennel, cardamom, mint, saffron.

For cooking – fennel, aniseed, turmeric, cinnamon, coriander, mint, liquorice, lemon grass, rose water, saffron, peppermint, dulse.

Movement

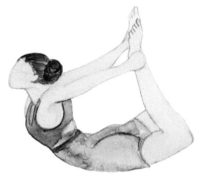

Pitta's should favour more relaxing styles with asanas including: Bow pose, a fantastic stretch for the abdomen improving digestion and bringing a fresh supply of blood to the lower organs to cool the pitta fire (Figure 3.)

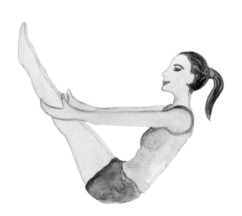

Half boat to tone and strengthen the lower back, buttocks and back of thighs (Figure 4).

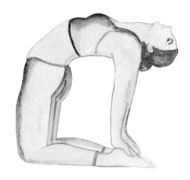

Camel pose opens the rib cage, lungs and digestive system, stimulates the thyroid and creates space to pacify excess heat and re balances the doshas (Figure 5).

Breath
The pranayama 'Breath of fresh air' technique helps purify and recharge both body and mind.

Massage
Best suited to more flowing rhythmic movements using a soothing oil blend to calm and relax the body.

KAPHA

Seasons
Increases in the Winter and lasts until early Spring.

Foods
Kapha needs to avoid comfort eating if feeling low and to avoid overeating and napping in the daytime, which will result in weight gain if not careful. Seek out foods rich in omega 3 fatty acids like fish, fish oil and flaxseeds, which help improve your memory at a time when you feel a little foggy, and replenish the body with anti-oxidant rich fruits and vegetables.

Herbs/Spices
For oily/clammy skin and to heat the body go for neem, sage, rosemary, triphala

For cooking – black pepper, chilli, ginger, mustard, nutmeg, cloves, bay leaves, allspice, cardamom, cayenne, marjoram, cumin, caraway, cinnamon, basil, anise, turmeric, sage.

Movement
With a tendency to over sleep and be somewhat sluggish, high impact exercise helps raise metabolism, boost natural release of endorphins and prime the body for action.

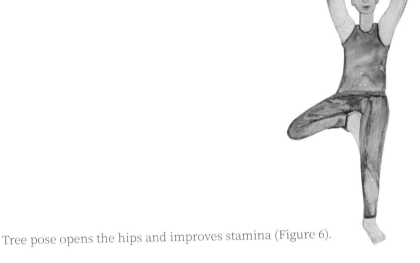

Tree pose opens the hips and improves stamina (Figure 6).

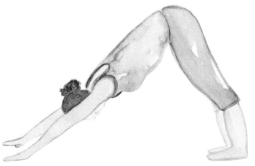

Downward facing dog helps expand the rib cage, chest and abdomen, and tones

the core and waist (Figure 7).

Breath

Controlled breathing, or pranayama helps regulate, rebalance and purify Kapha's internal energy.

Massage

Vitality-boosting movements delivered with an energising oil blend.

ΛCKNOWLEDGMENTS

Thank you to:

Satya, Kamlesh, Anju, Maneeshka, Kiren, David, Lanah and Lenni, my family.

Adrian Reynolds, my editor and wise counsel, this book would not be here without you.

Kate Patrick for helping me define my brand.

PR for Books, my PR partner.

Mia Alhabori, my cover designer.

Jo Welch, my photographer.

Anjali Puri, my illustrator.

Miranda Boscawen, Jenya Di Pierro, Julie Dent for your methods.

Davidji, Kate O'Brien, Dr Aseem Malhotra, Dominique Antiglio for your endorsements.

For now we are energy that matters.
While we are …
Be kind to self.
Be kind to others.
Be kind to planet
… before returning to the energies that birthed us.

ΛBOUT THE ΛUTHOR

"Whatever we do in life, we owe it to ourselves to be the best we can be"

Sunita Passi is a renowned specialist in Ayurvedic medicine, an award-winning skincare entrepreneur and a wellness visionary helping to shape an alternative future for healing and health.

Over a 20-year career in Ayurveda, she has trained over 1,000 practitioners and brought authentic, practical tools for natural health into the lives of thousands more. Her business model combines this passion for healing with environmentally and socially conscious practices and a clear-sighted focus on her higher purpose: to change the paradigm around wellness.

Sunita grew up in the midlands, UK and was first introduced to Ayurvedic medicine by observing her grandfather, Ayurvedic practitioner Dr Hazari Lal Passi, in his clinic in northern India. She later entered the field of investigative journalism, pursuing a fast-moving career that was a far cry from the gentle world of holistic healing. But the seeds had been sown.

At a certain point, Sunita realised that the path to human wholeness lay not in conventional medicine and hard-headed competition, but in adopting a mindbody approach that could be applied to every facet of one's daily lifestyle – looking to the ancient world to find inspiration and guidance for a better future.

This reconnection with her lineage as a healer proved a decisive turning point, and she quickly moved on from Ayurveda student to founding her own company, Tri-Dosha, in 2005. Tri-Dosha has now won multiple awards for its training programmes and hair and skincare products that draw on modern formulations with ancient herbal alchemies for their effectiveness.

Known for her fun, approachable and compassionate style, Sunita has become an articulate champion for natural healing, taking her message of treating the whole being out into a wider world. She has been a TEDx speaker, BBC Radio broadcaster, author and podcast host; she mentors students as an Alumni Fellow of Nottingham Trent University; and she coaches individuals and industry professionals through authentic wellness platforms, both online and in-person.